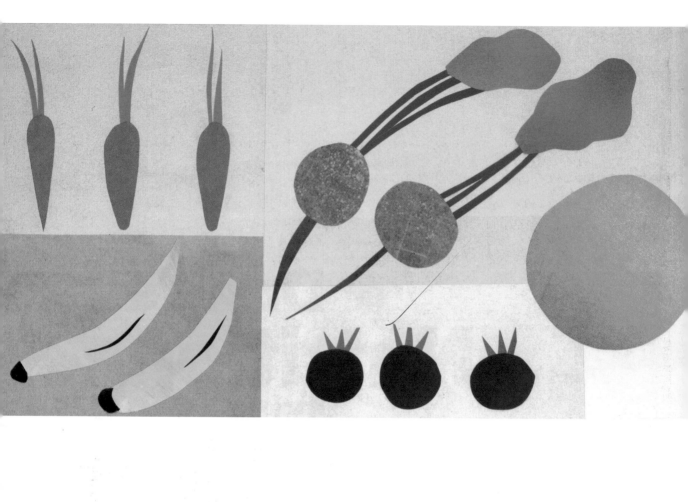

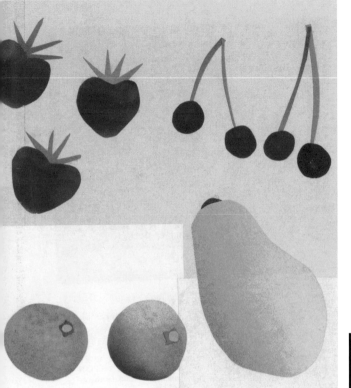

Dr Ali's
Nutrition
Bible

Dr Mosaraf Ali

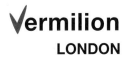

Vermilion

LONDON

To HRH The Prince of Wales
for his continuous support in
my work

First published in Great Britain in 2003

5 7 9 10 8 6

Text copyright © Dr Mosaraf Ali, 2003
Illustrations copyright © Sarah Jarrett, 2003
Design copyright © Vermilion, 2003

First published by Ebury Press,
Random House, 20 Vauxhall Bridge Road, London SW1V 2SA

Random House Australia (Pty) Limited
20 Alfred Street, Milsons Point, Sydney, New South Wales 2061, Australia

Random House New Zealand Limited
18 Poland Road, Glenfield, Auckland 10, New Zealand

Random House South Africa (Pty) Limited
Enulini, 5A Jubilee Road, Parktown 2193, South Africa

The Random House Group Limited Reg. No. 954009

www.randomhouse.co.uk

A CIP catalogue record for this book is available from the British Library

ISBN 0 09188 949 9

Illustrator Sarah Jarrett
Designers Maggie Town and Beverly Price
Editors Caroline Ball and Rachel Aris
Proofreader Claire Wedderburn-Maxwell
Consultant Nutritionist Fiona Hunter

Although every effort has been made to ensure that the contents of this book are accurate, it must not be treated as a substitute for qualified medical advice. Always consult a qualified medical practitioner. Neither the author nor the publisher can be held responsible for any loss or claim arising out of the use or misuse of the suggestions made or the failure to take medical advice.

Colour separation by Icon Reproduction
Printed and bound in Italy by Graphicom

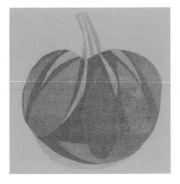
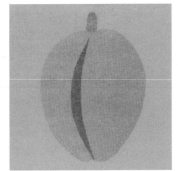
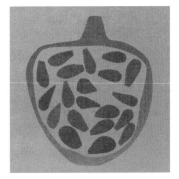

contents

introduction

As far back as I can remember, my mother was very strict about what we ate. Her father was a doctor and homeopath – a great example of an integrated physician – who firmly believed that diet, hygiene, exercise and sleep played important roles not only in preventing illness but also in building health, and he brought up his daughter to believe so too.

When someone in the family was ill their diet changed according to the type of illness. If any of we children should have diarrhoea, God forbid, our mother would feed us raw banana stew (a stool-binding dish), mushy rice and lots of salt and lime water to drink. She would boil the bark of the kashmala tree (rich in iodine, a powerful antibacterial) and mix the solution in goat's milk to temper it. If we had a fever, we would be given stir-fried patta (a bitter vine), sago or barley water with sweet lime juice for energy, and a cold compress on the forehead or abdomen to bring the temperature down, and told to rest in bed. We would have our throat massaged if it ached and inhale drops of mustard oil if our noses or sinuses were blocked. Whatever the ailment was, there was always a therapeutic diet that worked.

Growing up in India and learning from my mother and grandfather built a strong belief in me that diet is very important for the treatment of illness, but also that a healthy, well-nurtured body is less likely to succumb to illness in the first place.

My mother insisted that we had three meals a day eaten at proper times. Breakfast consisted of puffed rice cereal and milk with a banana. Lunch was normally vegetables, rice and fish or meat for protein. Dinner in the evening was always light – perhaps a lentil dish with rice and some vegetables. My grandfather said one should eat according to one's age and needs. Children needed more nourishing food than the elderly, and we were given more fish and chicken during examination periods as the brain needed more phosphorus and the body needed more protein.

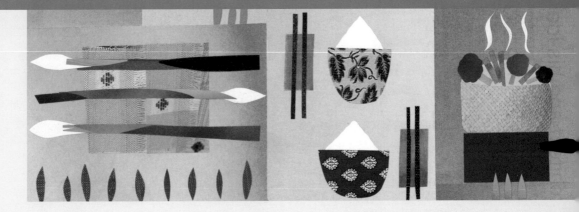

Against all the odds, the traditional regime continued at my boarding school – how the Irish and Australian Christian brothers were coaxed by their Anglo-Indian colleagues into introducing Indian methods of keeping children healthy will always remain a mystery. Every morning during the summer we had to drink a small glass of bitter chiretta brew to 'cleanse the blood', and once a month we were given a purgative of 'English salts' (magnesium sulphate) to clean the bowels, a ritual we all hated. It did, however, keep us healthy – very few children ever took sick or had diarrhoea (so common in India) and as teenagers we never suffered from pimples.

It was from this background that I spent many years learning and practising different forms of medicine around the world, and formulated my philosophy that we should draw the best from each. Numerous dietary traditions throughout the world have at their core a common-sense practice or acute observation that has been lost in a welter of ritual, or distorted as it has passed down the generations to become folk belief or an old wives' tale. Over the years I developed the Integrated Health Lifestyle Programme, based on Hippocrates' Regimen Therapy. The programme is fundamental to my work and I use it as a preventative measure and as the basis of all my treatment. This led me eventually to open my Integrated Medical Centre in London, where a team of registered medical practitioners covers almost every form of medicine and health practice.

Regimen Therapy rests on the tripod of diet, massage and yoga, on which health and well-being are established. These are all interdependent, but diet is at the core of them all – the wrong foods can fail to nourish us, can keep us awake at night, make us sluggish and overweight or tense us up, even poison us. Truly, we are what we eat.

But what should we eat? Food is big business and big news. Major food concerns, from BSE to GM foods, regularly hit the headlines, and almost every week another food story serves to confuse us further – broccoli reduces risk of stroke, red wine harmful, red wine beneficial, milk linked to Crohn's disease, curry hailed as new miracle cure, bacteria rife in organic chickens. What do we believe? With so many contradictions and confusions, what is the point of taking care with what we eat if we are likely to be told next month that it is all wrong?

Dr Ali's Nutrition Bible is all about understanding how different foods contribute to our health, and our ill-health. In Part One I begin with what food does for us, how our body processes it, which foods are good for us and which foods are bad. There is advice on food preparation and cooking, and the benefits of giving our digestive system a holiday from time to time.

From the theory I move on to the practicalities. We should never lose sight of the fact that each of us is unique. Diet is not a matter of 'one size fits all', and we should always strive to tailor our diet according to personal needs, and to change it as circumstances change. It is self-evident that a toddler, a lumberjack and an elderly woman all have different nutritional requirements, but dietary variations should be more subtle than that. So Part Two looks at food requirements at different stages in our lives, how to fit healthy eating into a variety of lifestyles, and the difference that genes and even temperament make. With the health MOT you can keep a regular check on how healthy (not how fit) you are, and what changes would make you healthier.

Part Three is concerned with how food and drink can help when things go wrong and we fall ill. This final part of the book is not an exhaustive prescription for every illness you might fall prey to – in fact it is my fervent hope that the guidance in Parts One and Two may mean you never need to read as far as Part Three! – but it is intended to help explain how nutrition fits into the overall picture of minimising illness and restoring health.

Following the advice in this book does not mean turning your back on conventional medicine – indeed about a third of the treatment carried out at the Integrated Medical Centre is 'conventional'. Instead, it should help with two things that hamper doctors and other health professionals but are within your power to change. The first is unhealthy patients. Taking greater responsibility for keeping your body in good running order is an effective preventative against many of the minor ills that fill doctors' surgeries; it will also help you heal more quickly and more completely if you do fall ill, relieving pressure on the demand for hospital beds.

Second is incomplete information. Treating an illness or disorder successfully depends on comprehending what has gone wrong – a diagnosis of the cause not just an analysis of the symptoms. And that needs the

> We should always strive to tailor our diet according to personal needs, and to change it as circumstances change.

understanding on your part that everything is interrelated, that how we lead our lives has a bearing on how our bodies will react to illness, how imbalances in one area cause strain in another, and that apparently unrelated symptoms can have a common cause. Telling half the story doesn't, in the long term, save a doctor's precious time and it can delay your recovery.

There are numerous books on nutrition, some based on the role of vitamins and minerals, some on calorie-counting, some on prescribed diets: food combining, macrobiotics, raw food, high protein/low carbohydrate plans and many others. I wanted to put together the facts about diet and nutrition that I learnt right from childhood and which I have recommended successfully to thousands of patients for over twenty years. I have worked in Africa, India, Russia, the Middle East, Hong Kong and Europe, discovering the rights and wrongs of eating habits all over the world, so although this book is aimed at people with a Western lifestyle, tastes and illnesses, it takes the best of what both West and East have to offer: a fusion of food, ideas and approaches to health that is truly integrated.

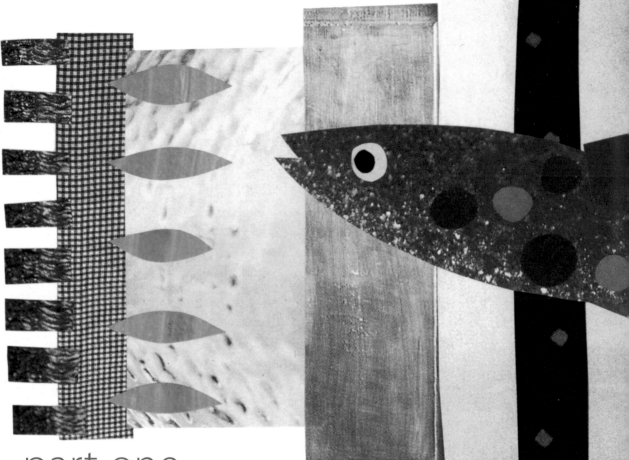

part one
eating for your body

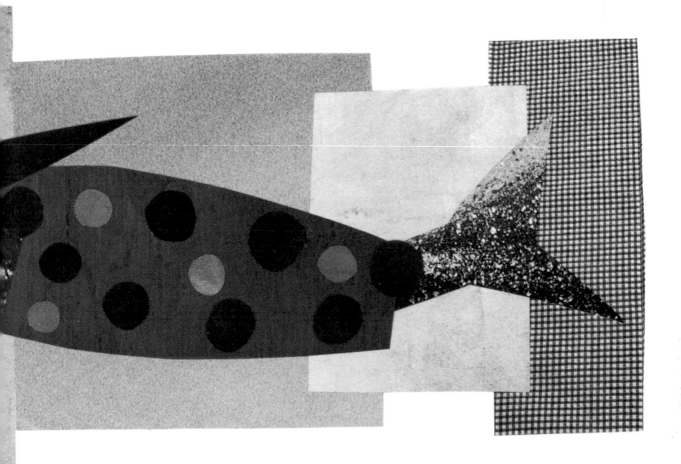

To be healthy we need to understand what is good for our body, how it reacts to what is bad, learn to read the signals our body sends us, and to adjust our eating habits as our body and our life changes. Like a business, a successful body needs good management to ensure happiness and productivity, and a well-run body should be a joy to live in.

chapter 1
nourishing your body

Imagine you are standing in front of a large dining table, and on it are all the foods you might eat and drink. Right in the centre are the main courses – lamb, beef, chicken, fish, shellfish, some highly spiced, some in rich, creamy sauces. Next to them are tureens of soups and platters of vegetables: peas and beans, artichokes, broccoli and salads. Beyond them are the desserts: cool sorbets, treacle pudding (and custard) and gâteaux.

On one side are wines and spirits, a range of liqueurs and aperitifs, and a good port. Next to them, perhaps some fruit juices – apple, cranberry, orange – and bottles of fizzy drinks. Then there is a variety of cheeses, bowls of nuts and crisps, and other snacks like biscuits, olives, some fancy canapés and a large chocolate cake. And don't forget the water, sparkling and still, and those staples, bread and potatoes. Quite a feast to choose from.

Now take a bucket. Go round and pick up the food you most like – and dump it into the container. Chop it all up small and mix it well. Pour on all the drinks you want, add all the chilli sauce and ketchup you like. Churn it all up and just look at it. Smell it. Look at the colour. Just imagine your system when

you dump all this on it at once! Why are we surprised when our bodies sometimes rebel?

The most obvious lesson from this is: don't overload your system. Respect that your stomach has a certain volume; don't overstretch it. Eat slowly. If you gobble your food it all arrives in the stomach in a rush, not properly chewed, resulting in excess work for the stomach, making it churn uncomfortably and produce too much acid.

If moderation is the key to a healthy body, so is diversity. The answer is not to cut down on the variety of foods that we eat as that is how essential nutrients get left out. Vary your diet to get all the vitamins and minerals you need, and you will have no need of supplements.

energy stores

It is the food we eat that gives us our energy. The most familiar way of measuring energy is in calories – when you consume energy you burn up calories, and when you eat you build up the supply. How much energy you require depends on many factors, such as your age, level of activity and the climate, but what is true for almost everybody is that if you regularly take in more energy (in the form of food) than you are expending, your body will store it as fat. The other side of the coin is that your store of energy is not unlimited. Put too much strain on the supply and you will tire; eventually, a system will fail.

Every cell of the body contains energy molecules known as ATPs (adenosine triphosphates). These can be moved freely throughout the body to supply energy where it is needed: to muscles for exercise, to the brain for thinking, to the intestinal tract for digestion and so on. The exact process is so far not fully known, but what is certain is that energy migrates all over the body and can be directed to the areas most needing it at any time.

Expending energy is not just physical. Mental work takes energy too and, although digestion may seem passive, it probably drains more energy from us than physical work does.

what is in our food?

The body requires six different types of food. The three building blocks are proteins, carbohydrates and fat. To that we add vitamins and minerals, which stimulate the enzymes and chemical reactions in the body. The sixth type is water.

As a rule of thumb you need around 60 per cent carbohydrates, 10–15 per cent proteins (depending on your activity level), 25 per cent fats, various minerals and vitamins and plenty of fluids, at least 2 litres or 6–8 large glasses of water a day.

carbohydrates

These provide us with energy, feed the brain, help control the breakdown of proteins and fight toxins. Most of the foods we eat that are not fat or flesh provide us with carbohydrates, but these vary widely, both in their nutritional value and the type of energy they provide.

Simple carbohydrates are more familiar to us as sugars. As well as sugar itself, we get these from honey, most fruit and some vegetables.

Simple carbohydrates are tasty and easily digested. They also provide us with a quick burst of energy (see page 44), but they should not form the basis of our carbohydrate intake. This should come predominantly from complex carbohydrates, or starches.

Complex carbohydrates are found in rice, noodles, yams, root crops including potatoes, bread, wheat and other grains, bananas and leafy vegetables.

Complex carbohydrates can be burned anaerobically, that is without oxygen, by producing energy molecules and lactic acid, which can be burned aerobically (with oxygen) later. This is why they are popular with athletes – that extra burst of energy, more than their oxygen supply can support, may mean the difference between winning or losing.

Carbohydrates also provide us with another essential element in our diet: **fibre**. Soluble fibre is gum-like (pectin, which makes jam set, is a form of soluble fibre) and tends to stick to potential waste

satisfying a sweet tooth

We all crave something sugary from time to time, but certain sweet foods are better for us than others. Sugars that are still an integral part of the food source are known as intrinsic sugars. Those that have been extracted from the food source are called extrinsic or free sugars. As foods are processed and become further removed from their natural state, fewer nutrients survive. For example, 2 teaspoons of white sugar (extrinsic) provide us with 48 calories and nothing much else. One apple, on the other hand, provides the same number of calories and contains about 12 g of sugar (intrinsic), but it also supplies useful minerals such as potassium, magnesium, phosphorus, iron and zinc, and nearly 2 g of fibre. So next time you fancy something sweet, try to reach for the fruit basket rather than the cake tin.

products and guide them out of the system. It is said to lower cholesterol levels.

Insoluble fibre, also referred to as roughage, absorbs water and adds to the bulk in the bowel. This eases the passage of waste and lowers the tendency for infection to build up. The bulk also tends to make you feel full. Most plants in our diet provide a mixture of soluble and insoluble fibre.

The table overleaf shows the approximate proportions of soluble to insoluble fibre in a range of foods. This is not how much fibre each food actually contains. Processed white breads and pastas have a greater proportion of soluble fibre, but have a much smaller overall fibre content. Wholemeal bread contains nearly four times, and wholemeal pasta nearly three times, as much fibre as their refined white equivalents. You can see that many fruit, especially dried fruit, have a greater proportion of soluble fibre (prunes are over 70 per cent fibre), while vegetables and some pulses are about half and half, and fibre in grains is more insoluble than soluble.

fibre content of common foods

	soluble	insoluble
apples		
raspberries		
apricots, cherries		
dried apricots		
plums		
prunes		
bananas		
mango, papaya		
almonds		
walnuts		
asparagus		
carrots		
cabbage/kale		
cauliflower		
potatoes		
French, runner beans		
peas		
red kidney beans, haricots		
lentils		
rice		
cornflakes		
porridge		
wholemeal bread		
white bread		
wholewheat pasta		
white pasta		

proteins

These are the body's building blocks. As well as building bones and muscles they support repairs, help in digestion and feed the immune system. We get our protein mainly from meat, fish, milk products, eggs, nuts and, in lesser concentrations, from vegetables.

You will often hear references to first- and second-class, complete and incomplete or high- and low-quality proteins. This refers to the amino acids they supply. Proteins from animal sources contain all eight of the essential amino acids that our body requires (hence first-class, complete etc.), but plant proteins are missing some of these. For this reason, vegetarians need to be careful about combining different sources of protein to avoid deficiencies (see page 36).

Few foods are purely one element, and most of our sources of protein also supply us with either carbohydrates (vegetable proteins) or fats (animal proteins). Meat and fish eaters are highly unlikely to be eating too little protein, but need to be wary of taking in too much fat with it: a lean pork fillet and a skinless chicken fillet will give you approximately the same amount of protein, but the pork contains nearly four times as much fat (although even this is only a fraction of the fat in a beefburger!).

fats

Fats are often considered the baddies of the diet, but we can't do without them. The body needs fat for growth and repairs, to regulate temperature and to cushion vital organs. They are a concentrated source of energy and contain vitamins A, D, E and K. Like carbohydrates, fats come in several types and most foods contain a mixture, but in different proportions.

Saturated fats tend to be solid at room temperature and are often our 'favourite' fats – cream, butter, cheese – but they raise cholesterol levels in the body (see page 16).

Trans fats, such as hard margarines and solid cooking fats, are used in many shop-bought cakes and biscuits. These are unsaturated fats but have undergone processing that causes them to act in our diet like saturated fats, and so are best avoided.

Unsaturated fats contain essential fatty acids. These are needed by our bodies to help fend off a variety of ailments, including heart disease and arthritis, and help lower cholesterol. They also contain vitamin E. These can be polyunsaturated or monounsaturated fats. Monounsaturated types have been found to have an even greater beneficial effect on cholesterol levels than polyunsaturated ones.

Food does not have to be fatty to provide fats: lean meat is sufficiently high in fats without needing to be supplemented by fatty cuts, and butter, cheese and cooking oils should be kept to a minimum. During the cold winter months our body needs more fat than in the summer.

fat content of common foods

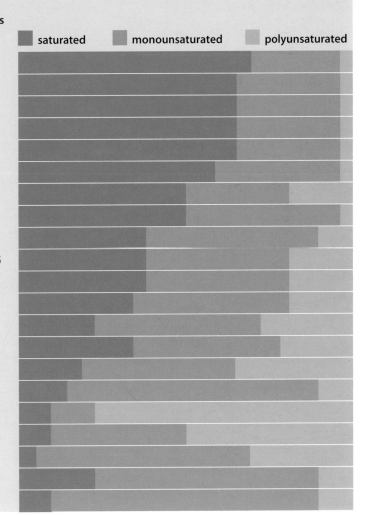

	total fats (%)	saturated	monounsaturated	polyunsaturated
butter	80			
cheddar cheese	34			
brie	26			
whole cow's milk	3.9			
double cream	48			
milk chocolate	30.8			
puff pastry	23.6			
beefburger	16.7			
roast beef	5.1			
pork sausage	35.25			
lean back bacon	6.7			
duck (without skin)	10			
mackerel	16			
eggs	16			
groundnut oil	100			
olive oil	100			
walnut oil	100			
blended vegetable oil	100			
rapeseed oil	100			
avocados	19.5			
hazelnuts	64			

cholesterol

There is much hype and concern over cholesterol; it is one of those trigger words, like 'calorie', that has become associated with 'bad', as if it wasn't needed. But, like calories, our bodies do need cholesterol – just not too much of it.

Our cholesterol comes from two sources: the liver, which releases some every day for the body to use in making, among other things, hormones and bile (this is blood cholesterol), and some foods (dietary cholesterol). Cholesterol is sometimes thought of as synonymous with fat, which it is not. The main reason for an increase in blood cholesterol, however, is saturated fats (see pages 14–15). Dietary cholesterol, confusingly, does not come mainly from high-fat foods. Principal cholesterol-rich foods are egg yolks, crustaceans (prawns, shrimps etc.) and liver and other offal.

A high level of blood cholesterol leads to the furring and blocking of the arteries (see page 172), but not everyone agrees about the contribution dietary cholesterol makes to blood cholesterol levels. In most people, the body does a great balancing act to ensure that fat in the diet doesn't have too great an effect on blood cholesterol levels. Genes play a large part here. Some people have a naturally high production of blood cholesterol, which means a diet that increases it even a little can raise the level unacceptably, while people with low natural production are much less at risk.

Genes can also be responsible in another way. Cholesterol is carried around in the blood on lipoproteins. These come in two types: low-density (LDL) and high-density (HDL). LDLs carry about three times as much cholesterol as HDLs, so a higher proportion of LDLs in the blood means a potentially greater amount of cholesterol. Genes are not the only things to affect the ratio of LDLs to HDLs. Exercise can help tip the balance in favour of HDLs, but being overweight favours LDLs. Hormonal balance is also a factor, which is why some metabolic disorders increase the proportion of LDLs, but women, especially before the menopause, are believed to have some 'natural protection'.

Foods that may help to control your cholesterol levels are:
• Garlic.
• Oats and oatmeal.
• Dried fruit.
• Fruit high in pectin, such as apples.
• Monounsaturated fats, such as olive oil.
• Soya beans (including soya milk).
• A moderate amount of red wine (1–3 glasses a week).

Having your cholesterol level checked periodically is a good idea, particularly if you have a tendency towards high blood pressure or have heart disease in the family. It is far better to take sensible preventative precautions such as reducing your saturated fat intake than to resort to cholesterol-lowering drugs.

vitamins

Vitamins are vital to our growth, development and continuing good health. Their roles vary from releasing energy from the food we eat and maintaining healthy hair and skin to helping the body to use other nutrients (vitamin D is vital to the absorption of calcium). Deficiencies can lead to serious illnesses, but an excess can also sometimes be dangerous.

Our body can store some vitamins but not others (the liver, for instance, can hold enough vitamin A to last for ten months). With those that cannot be stored there is little likelihood of taking in too much, since the excess is simply excreted. This also means, however, that we have to keep up a regular intake of these vitamins: it's no good thinking that because you have eaten two huge platefuls of cabbage and a dozen oranges that you won't need to take in any more vitamin C for a while.

It is easy to be misled into believing your intake is greater than it is. Green vegetables, for example, are a good source of vitamin C. But vitamin C decays with storage and leaches out into cooking water. So broccoli that has been in the fridge and then boiled will be considerably lower in vitamin C than steamed broccoli that was fresh from the garden.

a guide to vitamins

	role	good sources	notes
Vitamin A fat-soluble	Counters oxidants and toxic wastes; essential for the eyes.	Carrots, peaches, apricots, watermelon, green vegetables, liver and dairy fats.	Supplements not recommended unless a deficiency is diagnosed.
Beta-carotene fat-soluble	Generally regarded as a vitamin, as the body converts it to vitamin A	Carrots, mangoes, papayas, peaches (beta-carotene is responsible for much of red/orange colour in fruit and vegetables – broadly speaking, the richer the colour, the higher the level); also occurs in dark green vegetables.	
Vitamin B (see below) mostly water-soluble Group of 6 vitamins	Essential growth, the nervous system, digestion, metabolism and general maintenance.	See individual entries.	Sickness, stress, smoking and alcohol reduce levels in the body.
Vitamin B$_1$ Thiamin	Releases energy to brain and nerves in the form of glucose	Pork and bacon, nuts and many other high-protein foods.	
Vitamin B$_2$ Riboflavin	Helps maintain a healthy skin.	Dairy products and many breakfast cereals.	Deficiency often appears as a sore mouth.
Vitamin B$_3$ Niacin	Involved in the release of energy from food.	Meat, fish and many other foods.	Deficiency appears first as skin disease but can later affect liver. Excess can cause liver and kidney damage and affects blood vessels.
Vitamin B$_6$ Piridoxine	Metabolises protein and helps vitamin B3 release energy from amino acids.	Meat, fish, eggs, whole grains and a few vegetables.	Excess can cause nerve damage. There are strict controls on supplements containing B6.
Vitamin B$_{12}$ Cyanocobalamin The only B vitamin that the body can store	Essential to blood production and maintenance of nerves.	Animal and seafood products and seaweed.	Deficiency can lead to pernicious anaemia and nerve damage.
Folic acid and **Biotin** regarded as having affinity to the vitamin B complex	Folic acid plays a role in the formation of new cells, as in pregnancy. Biotin helps release energy from carbohydrates.	Wheat bran, liver, nuts, eggs and many other substances.	Folic acid, in particular, has upper safe level only twice the recommended, so supplements should only be prescribed by a physician.
Vitamin C Ascorbic acid water-soluble	Guards against cell mutations and premature ageing and helps prevent the oxidation of fatty foods. It supports the immune system.	Most fresh fruit and vegetables particularly the cabbage family, red and green peppers, potatoes, blackcurrants, strawberries, citrus fruit, tomatoes and amla (see page 178). Steadily lost during storage.	Deficiency results in poor healing of cuts, bleeding gums and nose, and a lowered immunity to infection.
Vitamin D fat-soluble	Vital for absorption of calcium and phosphorous, necessary for the maintenance and development of bones and other hard tissue.	Exposure to sunlight meets most needs. In sunless climates, or for people confined indoors, some dietary intake is necessary – animal fats, including dairy products and oily fish. Vegans are virtually dependent on sunshine or supplements.	Deficiency can appear as rickets in children, pain or weakness in muscles, bones and hard tissue in adults. Lack of absorption of phosphorus can lead to brain disorders. Excess can damage kidneys.
Vitamin E fat-soluble	Protects fats from oxidation and soaks up free radicals. Promotes healthy skin and prolongs life of red blood cells exposed to ultraviolet light (sun).	Fats, liver, green leafy vegetables, wheatgerm, nuts, corn oil.	High doses sometimes recommended as a supplement, but an excess can increase the risk of stroke.
Vitamin K fat-soluble	Essential in the clotting of blood.	Wide range of food, especially dark green leaves and fruit skins.	Deficiency very rare.

Most healthy people should be able to get all the vitamins they need from a good, varied diet, but requirements vary according to our age, sex and lifestyle: fast-growing teenagers, pregnant women, smokers (give up!) and the elderly are among the groups that may need to take extra care to ensure they are getting all they need (see Part Two).

minerals

Our bodies need inorganic chemicals derived from the earth in small but essential amounts to support the formation of bone, nails, teeth and blood cells. Micro-elements such as cobalt, copper, zinc and selenium, and minerals such as calcium, iron and magnesium are essential participants in different bodily functions, either directly or indirectly. A healthy, well-balanced diet is unlikely to leave you deficient in any of these, but there are some to take particular note of, or which hit the headlines from time to time and cause concern.

calcium

This is vital for bones and teeth, and for the functioning of muscles (which will draw calcium from bones if they have an insufficient supply). Good reserves of calcium help minimise the effects of osteoporosis in older people (see page 111). Various things, including lack of vitamin D, a poorly functioning digestive system, and tannin, interfere with calcium's absorption (see pages 16–17). Vegans and anyone who does not eat dairy foods need to ensure they get sufficient calcium from alternative sources.

GOOD SOURCES Found in abundance in many foods, especially milk (see illustration opposite) and cheese, but also dark green leafy vegetables like kale and spinach, seaweed and the edible bones of small fish (canned sardines etc.).

selenium

This mineral is necessary for a range of hormonal functions, from sexual development to the working of the thyroid. Selenium also contributes to the health of eyes, skin and hair, and is an antioxidant (see page 23). It has been in the public eye in recent years because of concern that wheat produced nowadays has a lower selenium content than in the past.

GOOD SOURCES Grain and also seafood, liver, meat, avocados, Brazil nuts and dairy produce.

iron

We require iron to manufacture blood, and deficiency is a common worry because it causes anaemia. Women are more prone than men to mild anaemia, especially when menstruating. Problems usually lie, however, not in too little iron – it occurs in a wide range of common foods – but in the inability to absorb and therefore make use of it. As iron is absorbed through the stomach, the problem is usually a form of gastric upset. Vitamin C helps take-up of iron from plant sources.

GOOD SOURCES Red meat, offal, spinach and broccoli, pulses and 'fortified' breakfast cereals.

sodium

This is the one mineral that we are all aware of eating, because ordinary table salt is sodium chloride. It occurs naturally in many foods, but we are also in the habit of adding it while cooking and sprinkling it over our food. We need sodium to regulate our bodily fluids and for our nerves to function, but unless you live in a tropical climate that makes you sweat a lot or you are consciously reducing your intake, you are likely to be eating too much rather than too little. Sodium in excess can raise blood pressure, increase anxiety, bring on insomnia by exciting the brain and exacerbate conditions like water retention. It can also cause skin irritations and interfere with the healing process. Sodium works in tandem with potassium and the two need to be kept in balance (see page 21).

GOOD SOURCES Found naturally in varying levels in meat, fish and vegetables, but is a common preservative and a flavour enhancer in prepared foods from soups and sauces to breakfast cereals.

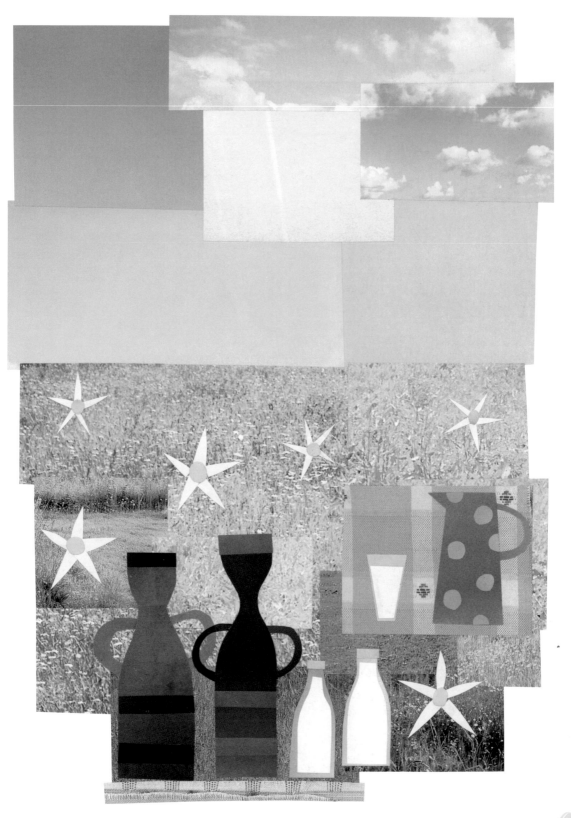

varieties of milk

Milk is rich in calcium and a useful source of several vitamins and minerals; it is a good source of protein for vegetarians, too. Once upon a time, milk meant fresh cow's milk straight from the udder. Now, however, we are offered a plethora of different types of milk: pasteurised, homogenised or UHT; milk from cows, goats or sheep; milk low in fat or high in calcium. What are the differences between them all?

Unless you live on a farm you are unlikely to come across milk that has not been **pasteurised**, i.e. heat-treated to kill disease-carrying bacteria. Milks given further heat treatment to increase their shelf life are described as **sterilised** or **UHT** (ultra-heat treated).

Full-cream milk is just under 4 per cent fat – in traditional milk bottles you can see the cream has risen to the top. **Homogenised** milk has been whipped so that the cream doesn't separate out. **Semi-skimmed** milk has had just over half the fat removed and in **skimmed** milk practically all the fat is removed. Skimmed and semi-skimmed milks retain the calcium and water-soluble vitamins of whole milk, but lose vitamin A, which is fat-soluble. This and the lower fat content is the reason that reduced-fat milks are unsuitable for young children.

Is **high-calcium milk** better for you than ordinary milk? No. Milk contains a natural balance of calcium and vitamin D, which is needed for the absorption of the calcium. Take in extra calcium alone and it will just pass straight through your system.

Lack of a particular digestive enzyme (lactase) in certain people makes it difficult for them to digest milk sugar (lactose). Symptoms include a bloated feeling, headaches, abdominal cramps, diarrhoea and catarrh and sinus problems from excessive mucus production. Young children also get skin rashes. This lactose intolerance is surprisingly common and many people suffer its effects without realising the cause. A simple remedy is often to switch to **goat's** or **sheep's milk**, or to soya milk.

Buttermilk has been churned to skim off the butter and is much more easily digested, making it a highly potent and beneficial drink.

Soya milk is not milk at all, but a milky-looking liquid produced by soaking soya beans. 'Fresh' soya milk (look for it in supermarket chiller cabinets) is much closer in taste to real milk than the long-life kind. Soya milk contains protein (being a pulse derivative) but lacks the fat-soluble vitamins of milk. It makes an acceptable alternative in tea and to pour over cereals but is nutritionally poorer in quality than real milk, so you will need to ensure you are getting the calcium and vitamins you need from another source, or buy calcium-enriched soya milk. See also pages 36–8.

Milk is a powerful antacid. Cold milk is often used to ease heartburn, and painkillers should be taken with milk, which will help soothe any irritation they may cause to the stomach wall. It is also recommended for many herbal medicines, especially those taken at night. Its ability to neutralise acid, however, means that drinking milk with a meal is not a good idea as it will interfere with digesting the food.

> Milk is a powerful antacid. Cold milk is often used to ease heartburn, and painkillers should be taken with milk.

> Milk is rich in calcium and a useful source of several vitamins and minerals; it is a good source of protein for vegetarians.

iodine

This is an essential component of thyroxine, which is produced by the thyroid to regulate the body's metabolism and mental development. Like selenium, the iodine content of vegetables and grains depends on the constitution of the soil in which they are grown (in regions where people are dependent on crops for their iodine but the soil is deficient, swollen thyroid glands – goitres – can be a common feature).

GOOD SOURCES Seafood and seaweed, iodised salts, yams, aubergines and jamun (an Indian berry).

potassium

Functions with sodium to send electrical nerve impulses to our brains, muscles etc. An increase in foods high in potassium will help counteract the effects of too much sodium, but as our diets are unlikely to be deficient in potassium, and an excess is unwise, it is better to maintain the equilibrium by lowering the sodium levels.

GOOD SOURCES Fresh fruit and vegetables, especially carrots, bananas, potatoes, celery, prunes, grapes, watermelon and avocados.

zinc

Vital to many of our body's functions and development (a deficiency will retard a baby's growth), zinc plays an important part in our immunity to disease. A slight deficiency can make you feel below par. Taking 15 mg of zinc every other day for a couple of months and then once a week will build up resistance to common infections such as coughs and colds. This can be increased to every other day during times of high risk, such as during the hay fever season (if you are susceptible) or over the winter months.

GOOD SOURCES Shellfish, meat and poultry, eggs; in smaller concentrations in grains.

cobalt

Important for blood synthesis – increasing your cobalt intake will correct a tendency towards slight anaemia.

GOOD SOURCES Fresh vegetables and fruit, especially pomegranates (which derive their colour from cobalt).

A deficiency in any mineral is bound to have an adverse effect on the body's normal function, but mineral supplements should be avoided unless your doctor has diagnosed a deficiency. The liver stores most minerals for long periods and any mineral in excess can be harmful to the liver, pancreas and heart (see also pages 23–4). Where possible, taking foods rich in a particular mineral is a healthier option than taking the mineral in isolation.

phytochemicals

Our forebears knew that many foods had distinct beneficial properties – mint to aid digestion, pineapple or papaya juice to tenderise meat, limes to ward off scurvy on long sea journeys – long before it was understood why. The latest discoveries to enlarge our understanding of what makes certain foods good for us are phytochemicals. Ongoing research is finding that these chemicals, found in vegetables and fruit, provide protection against a range of illnesses and infections from cancer to heart disease, and many of them act as antioxidants (see page 23).

Much has still to be learnt about the contribution of individual phytochemicals to our health, but the important thing to remember is that this is just giving scientific proof to the long-observed evidence that plenty of good-quality, organic fruit and vegetables are vital in our diet (see illustration page 22), and that certain foods are especially powerful in the fight against ill-health. It is also better to think of improving your diet by eating a variety of whole foods, rather than searching out extracts and specific phytochemicals.

There are many thousands of different phytochemicals, arranged into several groups, but you may hear in particular about:

Bioflavenoids help with absorption of vitamin C and also protect against cancer. One, quercetin,

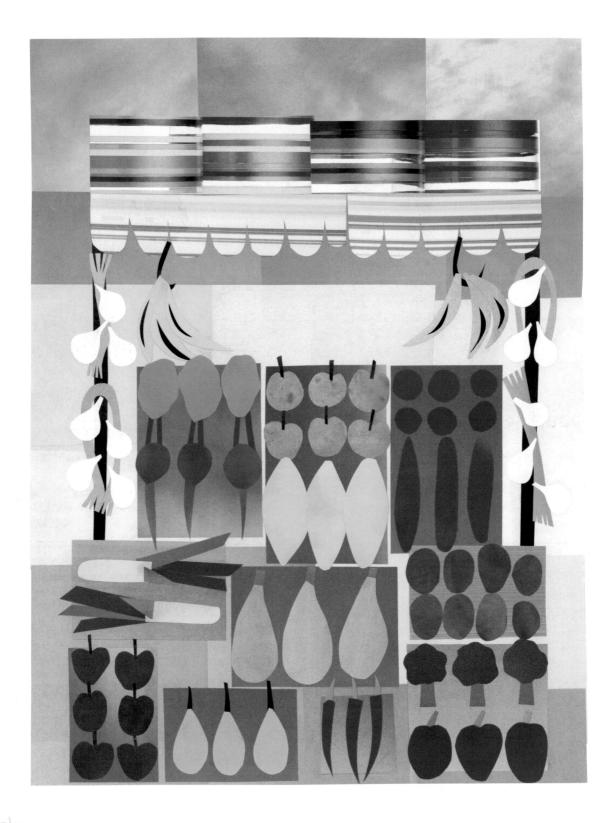

eating for your body

acts like an antihistamine (helpful for hay fever) and may also reduce the chance of cataracts in the eye; it is found in a variety of produce including apples, onions, potatoes and red wine.

Caretenoids include lycopene (from which red fruit and vegetables, especially tomatoes, get their colour), which may lower cholesterol and significantly reduce the risk of heart attacks and also protect against some cancers; and lutein, in blackcurrants and dark green leafy vegetables, another anti-carcinogenic. Beta-carotene (associated with vitamin A, see page 17) also belongs in this group.

Glucosinolates seem to help build up our body's defences against cancerous growths. The brassica family are excellent sources, especially Brussels sprouts and broccoli. Watercress, which is related, contains isothiocyanate, which may protect against the carcinogens in tobacco.

Allicin is an organosulphide, a component of the allium family – onions, leeks, garlic etc. – and is effective against several digestive-system cancers and also in preventing problems related to blood circulation such as high blood cholesterol, embolisms (blood clots) and heart disease. Garlic is particularly high in allicin.

Isoflavones are a type of phytoestrogen, helpful to women in reducing the effects of the menopause and also protecting against breast cancer. Pulses are the main source.

antioxidants

Our bodies naturally create charged particles called free radicals. These go around stealing electrons from healthy molecules. We can cope with a certain amount of this without problems, but if the free radicals multiply too much (caused by toxins in our diet and the environment) they start adhering to cells and causing damage, particularly to DNA.

Antioxidants absorb excess free radicals. Vitamins A, C and E and the minerals selenium, zinc and manganese, contained in fruit and raw foods, vegetables, soaked almonds and germinated seeds, are antioxidants. Many phytochemicals

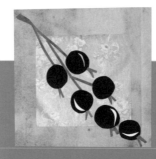

blackcurrants

These are very rich in vitamin C, a powerful antioxidant that helps to strengthen the immune system, prevent heart disease and aid the body's struggle against infections, cancer and arthritis. Blackcurrants retain their vitamin C content better than many other sources, even when cooked or preserved. The professor under whom I studied in Moscow used to boil dried blackcurrants in water for patients on prolonged fasts. He found the traditional lime and honey water too harsh for the fasting stomach, but blackcurrants provided vital vitamin C while keeping hunger pangs at bay.

are also proving to be effective antioxidants.

The argument for supplements is that natural antioxidant foods are lacking in essential ingredients by being grown in greenhouses or put in cold storage, destroying some of their nutritional value. There is some truth in this. They also suffer from the adverse effects of fertilisers and pesticides. However, the extent of this is not really known and it is possible to avoid it by eating organic fruit and vegetables. Generally speaking, if you don't put too many toxins in your body you won't need any extra antioxidants.

taking supplements

Today's fruit and vegetables tend not to be as potent as in the past thanks to the use of fertilisers and other chemicals. In many cases the soil itself lacks the minerals and micro-elements we need.

yoghurt and the power of 'friendly' bacteria

A healthy gut has a flora of 'good' bacteria that aid digestion and keep down 'bad' bacteria and fungal growth in the digestive system. If you take antibiotics over a long period they destroy the good bacteria along with the bad, and you are more vulnerable to fungal infections such as vaginal thrush, mouth ulcers and candidiasis (see pages 184–5 and 191). Gastric problems can also upset the balance.

A traditional treatment for a bacterial gut infection such as dysentery is to eat live yoghurt. Live yoghurt contains bacteria (lactobacilli) that aid digestion by breaking up proteins and carbohydrates to allow them to be processed and absorbed more quickly. They will also replenish the supply of 'friendly' bacteria. However, eating live yoghurt while taking antibiotics is a popular but false notion, as the bacteria mostly get killed off. The time to benefit from live yoghurt is straight after finishing the course, when it will quickly help to restore the balance. (Stir set yoghurt to maximise its effectiveness.)

In recognition of the effectiveness of maintaining a healthy flora of bacteria, foods that specifically contain a variety of active good bacteria are now available in yoghurt or milky form, or capsules.

Vitamins and minerals are essential to our bodies, so some supplements may be necessary. I do not, however, see the logic behind large doses of them, especially when the body's absorption power is good. As far as possible rely on natural sources, and maximise the nutrient value by choosing organically grown food and eating it as fresh as possible.

All dietary supplements should be treated with caution and are inadvisable unless work, disease and energy requirements demand it. Many of the vitamins and minerals that we ingest naturally through food are processed through the liver. The liver, endowed with great intelligence, will detect when enough of a substance has been received, and will excrete the rest (see page 29). However, many supplements are bio-engineered to bypass the liver and go straight into the bloodstream. In this way it is only too easy to take excess of a particular vitamin or mineral contained in a supplement, while this is very unlikely if taken naturally. Moreover, continuous intake of any potent substance makes the body immune to it, so you should take no more than you need and have gaps of a month or so between courses. It is a good idea to rotate them.

water
We need water for all bodily functions, especially elimination, and to regulate bodily temperature. It needs to be replenished on a continuous basis. In addition to the fluid contained in many foods, the body needs 2–2½ litres, or 6–8 large glasses of water a day. Drink water as you wish in between meals throughout the day, but don't drink significantly with meals, as I believe it dilutes the digestive juices.

tap water or bottled water?
Nowadays bottled water has become a big business as people do not like the taste of what is piped into our homes – see what we have come to: buying even this basic requirement for living. Barring accidents, tap water is hygienically safe, but it has been recycled many times and in many areas you can taste the chemicals used in its purification. Filtering it will remove residues and improve the taste.

Bottled waters vary widely in their mineral content and in their taste. Some have a natural sparkle, but most fizzy waters have been carbonated to give them their bubbles, and these can cause abdominal gas and bloating.

The curative properties of different spring waters have been known for centuries, and spas from Bath to Baden-Baden have thrived on people coming to 'take the waters'. Spring waters often cure ailments such as stomach ulcers, gastritis and chronic constipation, and there are springs whose specific mineral content is renowned for treating liver disease, anaemia, kidney stones and so on. Some waters have acquired deep religious or spiritual significance: the holy water of the Ganges (drunk by millions of people every day without major epidemics, despite its pollution), at Lourdes, and from the Zam Zam well near Mecca. Be it faith or the composition of the minerals, the waters seem to have some healing properties.

In my opinion, water that comes from deep in the earth has greater healing potential. These springs are long in contact with the minerals.

ringing the changes

• Many bottled waters come flavoured with orange, peach or other fruits. These flavours are chemical-based, so instead try flavouring water with a drop of vanilla extract or fruit juice.
• Fruit and herbal teas have seen a huge upsurge in popularity, from rosehip and chamomile to blackcurrant and mint. These are all ways of making your fluid intake more interesting, but vary them rather than sticking to one type. Herbs, even taken as teas, have powerful properties. Peppermint tea in excess, for example, can neutralise the acid in the stomach, but you need a certain amount of acid for digestion. Also, try not to sweeten these teas – your body can do without the added sugar or honey.
• Non-citrus fruit juices, like apple, cranberry, grape or pineapple are full of flavour, but dilute them as they are rich in fruit sugars. Differentiate between pure juice and 'juice drink', 'nectar', 'high-juice' and similar descriptions; these are usually high in sugar or sugar substitutes and sometimes have added colouring and flavouring.
• Tonic water would be excellent if it weren't for the added sugar (or sugar substitutes in diet tonics). It is a great neutraliser of excess stomach acid and helps curb hunger pangs. If you can find 'quinine water' without the other additives, drink it before a meal rather than after, when it will interfere with digestion.

Snow water that washes rocks or comes out of mountain springs may have a less pronounced taste, but may not have the right quality to heal stomach problems.

Do a taste comparison of different waters until you find one that appeals to your palate. Sip it on an empty stomach and you may be pleasantly surprised how your heartburn, indigestion or gas improves.

soft drinks
Other drinks have serious limitations. Most soft drinks and milk drinks are high in calories. Canned drinks are typically very high in sugar, often the equivalent of 2 tbsp per can. Some also contain nitrates. Energy drinks are potential hazards. Some contain caffeine, which will dilate blood vessels; you get an instant spurt of energy but you are tricking the body with chemicals. Some fizzy drinks have had the caffeine removed and replaced by other chemicals which have the same effect – but because they do not contain caffeine itself they can be marketed as caffeine-free. Read the ingredients!

Sometimes the ingredients list does not tell the whole story. Again, marketing hypes a 'secret formula' and a 'unique taste' whose source cannot be revealed. To get round the law manufacturers can add up to 20 different chemicals that need not be stated on the label if each is in sufficiently low quantities. Such small quantities could have a potent homeopathic effect far beyond the individual volume.

Chemicals are hard to avoid, even in our tapwater. Tapwater in most large cities is recycled. Efforts are made to check the bacterial content, the proportion of sodium and certain basic chemicals, but little is done to check its taste and other chemicals in small permissible doses. The body can deal with small doses, but the cumulative effect is worrying.

Alcohol suppresses the efficacy of the water it accompanies, as does coffee and to some extent tea (these are dealt with in more detail in Chapter 4).

chapter 2

a journey through the digestive system

The basic role of the digestive system is to process the fuel – food and drink – that keeps us alive and provides us with energy. A baby fed on milk grows incredibly fast, its body quickly and easily converting the milk into blood and flesh. Yet if you were to inject even a small quantity of milk directly into the bloodstream it would be asking for trouble, and might even prove lethal. We need the digestive system to convert what we eat into life-sustaining building blocks: glucose, amino acids, fatty acids, minerals, vitamins and so on. The first stage of digestion breaks down food particles mechanically or chemically, a process known as metabolism, or burning. The second stage absorbs the metabolised particles and the third stage then eliminates the unusable waste. Even though this sounds simple, it is a complex and well-coordinated process.

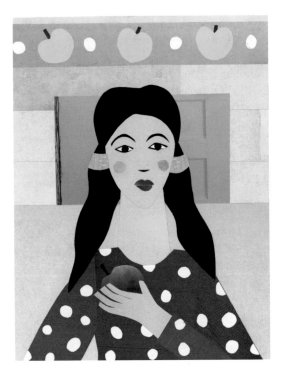

the mouth

Although the principal digestive processes go on in the gut, digestion begins in the mouth – or even before, since just the very sight or smell of something tasty can set our salivary glands in action.

If you eat very fast or do not chew properly, you bypass the first feedback mechanism that tells you when to stop eating and you will end up eating more than you should. This creates the first of many digestive problems – the sheer quantity of food puts extra stress on the system. Gulping down food creates a second hurdle for the digestive system. Overwhelmed taste buds are unable to send preliminary messages to the brain to prepare the correct mix of digestive juices to break down the particular food. Overloading a factory production line does not speed up production; on the contrary, it could gum up the works.

instant energy

Digestion takes time, but it is commonly known (and easily tested) that eating something sugary gives you 'instant' energy. How is this? As soon as the taste buds detect sugar in your mouth, they send a 'sugar' message to the hypothalamus (above the pituitary gland at the base of the brain), which passes it on, through the pancreas, to the liver. This triggers some of the body's stored sugar (glycogen) to be converted into glucose and released. So a chocolate bar or glucose tablet gives you a quick burst of energy and satisfies hunger pangs, not directly, but through the promise of replacing your own glucose reserves in your liver. The taste buds simply inform the brain that it is all right to release some glucose because more is on the way. Up to a point you can cheat this system by taking sweet-tasting substances (e.g. liquorice) to exhaust the reserves, until the body realises that it needs the real stuff.

the tongue

This is a highly specialised sensory organ. The nerve endings on the tongue (known as receptors) can identify temperature, coarseness of particles, moisture content (signalling salivary glands to secrete more or less saliva) and many other properties of which we may or may not be aware. These receptors are highly sensitive and they can identify every bit (physical, chemical, biological) of the particles or substances that enter the body orally. Homeopathic remedies in almost molecular dilution act on the receptors to powerful therapeutic effect. So sensitive are these receptors that, for example, the very presence of nuts in food can produce, in a person with a nut allergy, a catastrophic (sometimes fatal) anaphylactic shock. Significantly, the reaction starts soon after a nut is in the mouth, long before it is digested.

Taste buds identify the various types of food and inform the brain about the nature of the food that is coming in. They are designed to do qualitative analysis (sweet, sour, pungent, bitter, astringent, salty) and, if given a chance, some general quantitative analysis.

When allowed to do their job, taste buds not only allow us to enjoy food, but also give signals about the choice of enzymes necessary for easy digestion. So: eat slowly, chew well and let the food and drink have sufficient contact with the tongue.

The state of your tongue says much about your state of health (see page 131). Gargle and rinse it with water. Occasionally use gentle tongue scrapes or the teeth to keep the surface clean. Look after your tongue for other reasons too, as it has many roles – in swallowing, in sexual arousal (it is a powerful erogenous organ) and in signalling to the brain when the body is dehydrated. It is an important organ for producing physiological and emotional responses in the body – the pleasant, stress-relieving reaction to the first sip of a good wine or a properly brewed cup of tea is because of your tongue's sensitivity.

the teeth

Teeth are designed to cut and grind food to a coarse pulp. This makes digestion easier and helps avoid the problem of the stomach producing excess acid.

Teeth also have fine nerve endings and participate in 'sensing' particles. When a tooth's enamel is eroded, we are sharply reminded how cold or hot water, or something acidic like lemon juice, feels on the teeth. Those who have dentures or implanted artificial teeth know only too well that it 'doesn't feel the same'. Food doesn't 'feel' or taste as well as it should, despite a degree of adaptation. Even though the replaced teeth are perfectly matched, the lack of nerve-endings under the enamel means a loss of sensation, a bit like walking on artificial limbs. This affects the digestion as well. Looking after your teeth is therefore a good investment (see page 180).

saliva

The salivary glands opening into the oral cavity help soften food particles to make swallowing easier. They produce moisture and some basic chemicals, called enzymes, to start limited digestion. Chewing your food allows the salivary enzyme, ptyalin, to release small amounts of simple carbohydrates. This initial digestion releases some 'fuel' to the body immediately and quietens hunger pangs. Lack of saliva (as in Sjogren's disease) makes eating dry food such as bread, biscuits or meat extremely difficult.

Chewing gum, betel nuts, intoxicating herbs or tobacco upsets the salivary glands and puts a lot of stress on them. Chewing without eating causes more saliva to be secreted and excess saliva secretion means the enzymes may not be as potent. Saliva is already a very weak alkaline and the stomach acid will destroy it. Chewing like this before a meal is particularly to be avoided, as it overstretches your taste buds and much of the taste of the meal is lost.

the stomach

From the mouth, food and drink journey down the throat and oesophagus into the stomach. The stomach does not have the capability to digest food fully or absorb the nutrients. It is like an ante-room where materials are received, stored and prepared for digestion. Its various parts are designed to carry out specific functions like churning, mixing with acid and rotating (not unlike a washing machine), secreting digestive enzymes and, finally, storing the pulped food mass until it is time for it to move on.

Enzymes break up protein, fat and carbohydrates into digestible particles. The stomach does have a limited capacity to absorb some substances, such as alcohol, aspirin-like medicines and iron. Babies' stomachs have an enzyme, renin, that can digest milk, but in adults the stomach's acid just curdles milk (rather like lime juice or vinegar does). Iron is absorbed by the stomach, which is why upsets to the stomach's function, such as severe gastritis and surgery, cause anaemia. The stomach also absorbs alcohol, and bubbly alcohol gets absorbed more quickly, which is why champagne, or spirits mixed with soda water, make us heady quickly, especially on an empty stomach. Fats decelerate the process, as alcohol is fat-soluble, but give a heavy feeling – fats in the stomach can slow down its evacuation.

the journey along the intestines

The partially digested pulp in the stomach is highly acidic and could burn the intestine walls if released all at once, so the stomach releases its contents in small portions into the **duodenum**, the first part of the small intestine. Here, large amounts of alkaline mucus neutralise the acid before any damage is done. The gas produced by the reaction between the acid and the alkaline is the cause of bloating shortly after eating. It is also a major symptom of IBS (irritable bowel syndrome, see pages 150–54).

The main process of digestion and absorption now begins, as bile from the gall bladder and enzymes from the pancreas join secretions from the duodenum itself to break down the food.

the gall bladder and the pancreas

The gall bladder is a reservoir for bile, which is highly alkaline and counters the acidity of the stomach contents newly arrived in the duodenum. How much bile is secreted will depend on the quantity and acidity of what the stomach has released, but there is a limit to how much bile the gall bladder can secrete. The liver creates bile from aged red blood cells, but to destroy more than its quota would lead to anaemia. If you eat large quantities of foods, especially acidic foods, or if the stomach produces a lot of acid, the duodenum will not be able to take it all and the food mass will stagnate in the stomach – a major cause of discomfort and indigestion ('heartburn' is acid regurgitating into the gullet (oesophagus) and throat and then trickling down into the windpipe and lungs to cause severe burning).

The pancreas secretes enzymes that complete the digestion of carbohydrates, protein and fats. Its best-known role is in the secretion of insulin, a hormone that regulates the amount of glucose in the blood. A malfunction in the production of insulin results in diabetes (see pages 156–60).

the liver

This is the next most intelligent organ of the body after the brain. It acts as both a chemical factory and a warehouse, and has over 200 functions. It has more blood than any other organ, holding as much as half a litre at a time. As well as an arterial blood supply feeding the cells, as in every organ of the body, it has a venous blood supply from the intestines that transfers the nutrients absorbed from food.

One of its main tasks is detoxifying the blood. If everything we ate or drank entered straight into the bloodstream, bypassing the liver, we would be poisoned instantly. The liver converts digested food into products useful to the body. It metabolises carbohydrates and protein into energy and growth, discarding the waste. It stores glycogen in large quantities, to produce glucose as a reserve source of energy when we need it. If glycogen levels are insufficient it can synthesise glucose from protein.

When we ingest excess sugar or protein and the liver cannot cope, or does not need either of them, then it converts them into body fat. So eating too much sugar can lead to fatty deposits in the body. The cholesterol that the liver synthesises helps build cells or is used to make hormones. The excess is either converted into bile or deposited in the walls of blood vessels (see page 172).

The liver also metabolises protein, to be used later as an energy source. Some is used to make blood or to transport substances to the various tissues, such as iron to the bone marrow.

The liver can store enough vitamin D to prevent its deficiency for about four months, sufficient vitamin A to last the body ten months, and vitamin B_{12} for a year. It also stores iron and many trace elements such as zinc, magnesium and cobalt. Eight of the thirteen substances that help the blood to clot are manufactured by the liver, which is why excessive bruising is a symptom of liver disorder.

Another feature of the liver is that it is the main organ that neutralises and excretes poisons, drugs and hormones. On a week-long course of antibiotics you would accumulate a lot of problems if the liver were not able to eliminate the excess antibiotic.

absorption

Once the acidity of the food pulp has been neutralised and it has been thoroughly mixed with bile from the gall bladder and the digestive enzymes from the pancreas, it continues along the rest of the **small intestine** (first the **jejunum**, then the **ileum**). This long tube (about 6 metres (18 feet) in all) is full of folds, producing a large surface area in a compacted space. The lining of these folds have numerous micro-projections, called **villi**, which absorb the final products of digested food.

Proteins are broken down into smaller and smaller units until they are converted into amino acids. Carbohydrates are similarly processed to form glucose. Both are readily absorbed by the villi's blood vessels and transported to the liver. Fat, however, takes a different route.

Once reduced to a frothy soap-like mass by bile, fat is attacked by pancreatic enzymes to form fatty acids. These are then converted into microscopic droplets of oils (called chylomicrons) which are absorbed, not by the blood vessels of the villi, but by the lymphatic vessels of the villi. They are then transported by the lymphatic system directly into the major blood vessels emerging from the heart. Some fats, such as triglycerides, are useful, but others form plaque on the arterial walls, which can build up to dangerous levels (see page 172). The liver cannot destroy or store this fat because the blood carrying it only passes through the liver after it has been through the heart, leaving its deposits on the way. The fat-soluble vitamins, A, D, E and K are also dissolved in these droplets and so transported directly to the blood.

The final part of the journey is along the **large intestine**, or colon. Much of the usable material has already been absorbed, but some minerals, including calcium, magnesium and zinc, are largely absorbed by the colon. That is why chronic constipation or diarrhoea causes mineral deficiency. If the **colon** is too dry (often through constipation) it can result in complications like diverticulitis (see page 149) and piles (see page 141). When the body has extracted all it can from the food, it expels the waste as faeces.

chapter 3
eating well

We quite obviously need food to live, but does how we eat and when we eat, as well as what we eat, make a difference? Cows seem to eat all day every day, while crocodiles only eat once a week and pythons go for a month or even longer between meals. What did nature intend for us?

eating for energy and energy for living

The most common digestive problems are heartburn, acidity, burping, indigestion, food stuck in the stomach, excessive bloating, irregular bowel movements and stomach cramps. These are often brought about by overeating and are connected to the amount and mixture of food we eat.

Anything you can do to relieve the strain on your digestive system is helpful. A healthy digestive system means you extract optimum nutrition from your food and you are not devoting an unnecessary amount of energy to processing it. This will leave you feeling better and more energised for working more effectively and enjoying life.

Babies have a high metabolic rate (meaning they 'burn up' and convert food into fuel more quickly) and tremendous growth requirements, so they need to eat often. By the time we reach adulthood we have done all our growing, and the food we eat is for our body's maintenance. It manufactures new blood (completely replacing our blood every 125 days); the lining of the gut is also replaced, and our skin, hair and nails keep on growing. We also need a basic amount of energy to sustain life – for the heart to beat, the lungs to pump and so on.

But life is carried on at much more than this bare minimum. The rhythm of our lives, rather than that of our bodies, dictates that we need good doses of energy to see us through our work and social lives. That is why the concept of three meals a day arose: one to start off the day, one to replenish lost energy and see us through the afternoon, and another to keep us going for the rest of the evening.

biorhythms

Internal body clocks keep rhythms that regulate us daily (sleep), monthly (menstruation) and seasonally. They have been best researched by the Chinese, according to whom every organ has its own energy and system. If we look at the biorhythm of the body we see that the stomach and the small intestines are most active between 1 and 3 pm. So that is the time when they can perform best. They are at their lowest energy twelve hours later, between 1 and 3 am. Pulse diagnosis reveals that someone with an empty stomach around 8 pm has ceased activity in the stomach and the intestines. So if you eat a heavy meal about 8 or 9 pm, you force your stomach to be active against your body's natural rhythm.

The liver, on the other hand, is most active between 1 and 3 am, and the gall bladder between 11 pm and 1 am. Most people who get gall bladder colic suffer at this time, and most people who die of thrombosis, when the liver manufactures all the clotting enzymes, also do so in the middle of the night. The danger of deep vein thrombosis (DVT) on long flights may also be greater at night for this reason.

Our biological clock intends us, therefore, to make our major digestive period in the middle of the day.

replenishing rest

Digestion, although it may seem trivial, is a strenuous activity and puts tremendous demands on the body. Imagine the effort for the stomach of reducing tough fibres, meat or nuts to a fine pulp without the aid of a hard grinding surface like metal, plastic or even teeth. Think about the power the body expends in converting and absorbing food, both chemically and physically. Because these movements are involuntary, however, we are not conscious of this effort and tend to ignore it. It is, nevertheless, heavy-duty work.

Restful, undisturbed sleep each night allows the body to relax and recuperate, and this should include our hardworking stomachs. Muscles have to spend time in a state of complete relaxation (atonia) so that lactic acid and waste products can be effectively removed. The brain, which has been active throughout the day, needs the body to sleep so that it can rest (and lying down allows more blood to flow into the head, so dozing in an armchair is not ideal). It is during this time that vital organs such as the liver, and all the chemical reactions in the body, do much of their work.

Resting after lunch allows your body to divert its energy to the stomach's churning and processing, but sleeping or resting immediately after dinner in the evening can cause problems. Your diurnal time clock is telling you that now it is time to sleep, to relax completely, but your stomach is receiving

> ## Restful, undisturbed sleep each night allows the body to relax and recuperate.

contradictory orders, to start work on a mass of new food. A heavy dinner may mean discomfort and insomnia. To stimulate your stomach into working at a time when it is not normally active, take a walk or do some light physical work and allow at least a couple of hours, preferably more, between eating and going to bed – the time you go to sleep may be later but you are more likely to have an undisturbed night and wake refreshed.

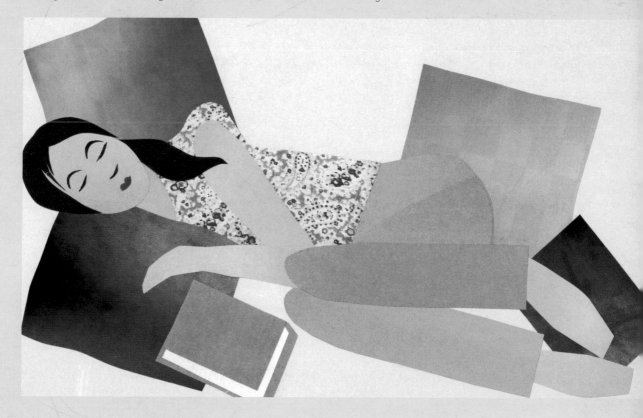

three meals a day

Where traditional ways of life are still maintained, the midday meal is the principal meal and dinner is light and taken early. Modern lifestyles often dictate, however, that we eat our main meal in the evening. A quick, unsatisfying lunch, or perhaps no lunch at all, means you are very hungry by the end of the day.

During the day you are usually active, so breakfast gets utilised, lunch gets utilised, but dinner does not. Many people eat a light breakfast because they have had a heavy dinner the night before. This is the wrong way round. Breakfast should be moderate. Lunch can be a good meal, but dinner is the one when most of the food gets absorbed but not used and causes problems with weight and digestion.

If you are going out dancing, to a party, playing tennis or squash after work, or going to swim or the gym, you will need a late boost of energy. More often, the evening is a time to relax, perhaps have some alcohol, spend time with the family, unwind from the day's exertions or stresses. It's a time when you are not worried about feeling sleepy or drowsy after the meal. Dinner has therefore become traditionally a heavier meal. This is satisfactory from a social point of view, but it is not health-orientated; it is an adaptation to the circumstances in which we work and live. We can condition our bodies to this, but it goes against the natural biorhythm.

phased digestion at night

A meal takes up to four hours to digest, and as our body's optimum time to digest food is during the early afternoon, by late evening it is not geared up to digest more than a certain quantity. Imagine you have eaten a big meal in the evening. For four hours the digestive system is hard at work. Then there is a lull. The muscles are exhausted, the stomach walls are exhausted, the gall bladder has been completely emptied, so it cannot carry out any more work. Everything comes to a rest. So an excess lies, only partially digested, in your stomach.

After a few hours' rest your body realises there is a lot of food left in the gut and begins work again. You may be woken from a deep sleep by the stomach's activity. You feel tired. Your bladder is full from the evening's digestive activity and you feel dehydrated because your body is drawing on fluid supplies to process and absorb the rest of the food. Your heart rate goes up with the effort. Your body is in turmoil. By early morning it is forced to concentrate on digestion rather than preparing itself for storing and releasing more energy.

Perhaps keeping you awake is nature's way of using some of that energy to digest all the food you forced yourself to eat, but a late dinner is providing energy that is not used. So it is stored as fat. Most people who habitually eat late dinners will have weight problems.

To eat heavily and late also leads to sleep disorders. Alcohol may send you to sleep initially but then dehydration or discomfort will wake you up. Regular disturbance will lead to problems not only of the digestive system, but also of the nervous system (see pages 204–7).

If you can, finish your evening meal by 7 pm. If you have had an afternoon siesta (see page 97) you are likely to be less tired and go to bed later, so dinner can be later too. But it should still be a light meal. Try to plan all celebrations to take place over the weekend – feasting and drinking during the week not only affects your digestion but also your energy levels, and thus your ability to function. Adrenalin will carry you along to a certain extent, but the problems will still potentially be there.

In circumstances where you have no control over the timing of your eating or your activities, you have to adjust in other ways. Try to keep your meal light and easily digestible, and avoid going to bed soon after eating. One of the things I recommend is a walk after dinner. After lunch, digestion is triggered by the body's natural biorhythm, but responses to a late meal will be sluggish. A walk mimics physical work, sending messages to the brain that you will be drawing on energy reserves and so it is time to activate the digestive system.

The gentle exercise will also help the stomach to churn food. Once the stomach is activated then it will continue the process.

Another useful digestion stimulant after a meal is adopting the Blessed Pose (*Bhadrasana*) for 5–10 minutes. This restricts blood flow to the legs, concentrating it in the abdominal region. See page 68.

listening to your body

How much we eat is influenced by much more than how much energy our body requires: habit, how our appetite is stimulated, how fast we eat and what we eat when.

take time to eat

As far as possible, sit down to eat. Do not eat in bed, lying down or semi-reclining, unless, of course, you are too sick to get up. Breakfast in bed seems like a luxury but it is bad for digestion. Your digestive system is designed to work best in the upright position, as some of our digestive process is aided by gravity.

So many people are in a constant rush and eat on the move, encouraging the pernicious habit of eating fast food fast. If you walk around as you eat a sandwich, or worse still something tougher to digest, like a hamburger, you are dividing your energy, putting unnecessary strains on the system. Of course you can walk and chew, but your appreciation of taste and therefore the early stages of digestion will be diminished. Appreciating your food properly is more satisfying, helps the early stages of digestion and makes it less likely that you will overeat. Even water, with its important minerals, should be savoured. Sit down, concentrate on enjoying your food and you will be less likely to eat too much too fast. Eating slowly is one of the keys to losing excess weight.

stimulants, suppressants and false messages

How hungry we feel is greatly swayed by how our appetite is awoken. Foods that increase stomach acid secretion generally stimulate appetite. Traditional 'tonics' used as pick-me-ups for people who weren't eating well were concocted from citrus fruit and alcohol. Nowadays people generally have too much stomach acid: stress, spicy food, alcohol, painkillers and canned products all add to the excess acid problem and stimulate our appetites inappropriately (see pages 40–41).

appetite stimulants	appetite suppressants
citrus fruit, pineapple	melon, dates, figs, peanuts
pickles	boiled or very bland food, such as puffy rice (absorbs acid)
chilli, ginger, garlic and spices; also some herbs (especially thyme)	chives and bitter leaves
cheese	fried and oily food
wine, champagne	bitter drinks (cranberry juice, tonic water, bitter beer) and carrot juice
enticing colour, attractive presentation	bulky food
smell of coffee and chocolate	sugar and sweet things

Stodgy, bland food and food with a lot of fat in it creates a feeling of fullness very quickly and stays in the stomach for a long time, deadening the appetite. You can often detect counterbalances to this in traditional accompaniments to fatty food. The Chinese, for instance, drink a lot of tea during an oily meal to flush away the fat. Similarly, serving mustard and horseradish with roast beef is more than just about taste – mustard stimulates acid, while horseradish stimulates bile, each aiding the digestion of the meat. (In the same way, tartare sauce and garlic help digest fish.) On the other hand, a chef cooking for large numbers at an Indian wedding or feast will add a lot of ghee to the rice dishes and the sweetmeats so that guests will quickly feel full and eat less, ensuring there will be enough food to go round.

Ayurvedic medicine identifies six tastes: sweet, sour, bitter, salt, astringent and pungent. To achieve variety, your daily diet should encompass all six tastes but distributed throughout the day, so as not to interfere with each other and send false messages to the brain.

As sweetness suppresses digestive action, sweets should generally be separated from other foods. Eating something sweet just before a meal ('I just must have a bar of chocolate to keep me going!') disrupts your digestion, because your brain has already got the false message that you have eaten (the brain has received the glucose it wants).

Pungent, astringent and salty food can produce the symptoms of dehydration, making you drink more water with your meal than you need.

Food that is bulky but without many nutrients also sends a false message. A watery vegetable broth, for example, will quickly stretch the stomach walls and so a 'full' message will be sent out to the brain's appetite centre in the hypothalamus, which will suppress further appetite. Further analysis, however, will reveal that there is little goodness to be had in all this liquid, and you will soon feel hungry again.

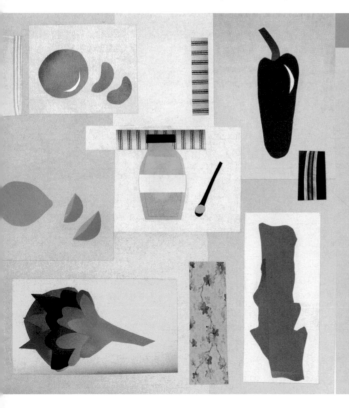

the six tastes of Ayurveda

According to Ayurvedic principles, foods can be categorised according to one of six tastes – sweet, sour, bitter, salty, astringent and pungent. Good health depends on balancing these six tastes in your daily diet.

Sweet: cherries, nectarines and sugar.
Sour: oranges, lemons, limes and grapefruits.
Bitter: chicory and artichokes.
Salty: smoked fish, table salt and seaweed.
Astringent: mustard and vinegar.
Pungent: chillies, peppers and ginger.

food combining

Different foods take different times to digest. Meat and fat can take at least two hours, and up to four hours, to be processed, while most vegetables take up to two hours; sugar and fruits are usually digested in just one hour. Puréed food presents a greater surface area for the enzymes to work on and is therefore digested more quickly. Boiled food also digests quickly, while raw fish and meat (like sushi or steak tartare) take longer.

Foods also have different chemical as well as physical constituents. Just imagine what happens when you mix coffee with ice cream (most commercial ice cream has a lot of bicarbonates and other chemicals as preservatives), then stir in an alcoholic liqueur. A chemical mixture like this would put a strain on the digestive system, but this is just what you might do at the end of a meal.

Out of these observations has developed the idea of food combining, which means constructing meals of food types that don't make conflicting demands on the digestive system. Vegetables and animal proteins combine well, starchy carbohydrates (pasta, potatoes, rice, bread etc.) combine well with vegetables, but carbohydrates and proteins clash and fruit is better eaten on its own. Many people have found it very successful for weight loss and accommodating different aspects of digestive health.

To avoid presenting your stomach with too great a mixture at once, you should generally eat more frequently. A little and often should be interpreted as a little of different things often, not more of the same. For example, don't eat a sandwich and have another an hour later. Use the breaks to separate out, in particular, foods that are mostly protein and mostly carbohydrate. Then the body can digest and cope with things much better. The regime I recommend is:
• Carbohydrates (cereals/porridge) in the morning.
• Protein with vegetables for lunch.
• Carbohydrates with vegetables in the evening.

Having a lighter combination at the end of the day is easier to digest and so less likely to be

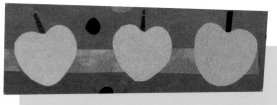

apples

Apples are nature's top fruit – one bite changed the whole consciousness of Adam. The skin (particularly of red apples) is rich in beta-carotene, iron and pectin, a soluble fibre that eases bowel movements. The pulp of green apples is rich in vitamin C and fructose, which gives them their sweet–sour taste. The enzymes in apples help digest protein. Commercially grown apples are often waxed to retain moisture and extend shelf life; wash this off thoroughly with hot water.

troublesome in the night. However, protein + carbohydrate forms the basis of many traditional meal combinations in the Western diet – think of fish and chips, ham sandwiches, bangers and mash, shepherd's pie, as well as familiar imports such as meat curry and rice or chicken and noodles. Overcoming this may seem daunting, but in fact, a shift in emphasis is often all that is needed. Food combining does not entail a complete ban on mixing protein and carbohydrates on the same plate, but recommends minimising one in favour of the other. A few tips:
• In a traditional meat-and-potatoes meal, substitute non-starchy root vegetables or pulses for the potatoes: try baked pumpkin or a spicy mash of red kidney beans.
• Add chickpeas or dried beans to a casserole instead of potatoes or barley.
• Choose vegetable (including salad) fillings for sandwiches and to accompany rice and pasta, rather than eggs, fish or meat.
• Pulses and lentils are high in both protein and carbohydrates, so can be combined with both.

• Salads and fresh vegetables similarly do not 'fight' with either proteins or carbohydrates in the digestive system. In fact, eating raw salad with meat or chicken aids its digestion.

• Allow at least four hours between a protein-rich meal and a carbohydrate-rich meal.

• Snack on fruit or vegetables rather than fats and starchy carbohydrates like bread and cheese.

• Fruit is best consumed as a titbit between meals, and better earlier in the day.

• Try to avoid eating food that takes a short time to digest very soon after food that takes a long time to digest. The effect will be to delay the quickly digested food from proceeding to the intestines for the nutrients to be absorbed.

vegetarianism

A vegetarian diet is often viewed as a healthy one because it usually means that you eat more fresh vegetables and fruit, more pulses and little in the way of saturated fats. Limiting the range of what you eat, however, means you need to make an extra effort in maintaining variety and interest in what you eat, and to ensure you do not put yourself in danger of missing out on certain vital nutrients.

Vegetarianism is quite a broad umbrella, covering a straightforward meat-free diet to eating only food of plant origin (veganism). These shades of meaning make quite a difference to your diet, so it is useful to look at what you are not eating, and then work out what alternative you need to include in your diet to compensate.

no meat

Fish and eggs will still be providing you with all the essential amino acids, and your diet will probably be lower in saturated fats (which is good news), unless you fall into the trap of replacing meat with a lot of high-fat dairy produce such as cheese.

good sources of protein for vegetarians

In combination and variation, the following foods provide the wide range of amino acids necessary to help the body synthesise its own (animal) protein. A good digestive system, proper preparation (soaking, germination, crushing nuts into powder form) and thorough chewing helps break these vegetarian protein chains into smaller ones that can be easily absorbed as amino acids.

• Almonds, soaked for 24 hours, and other kinds of nuts, especially Brazil nuts, walnuts, hazelnuts, pecans, chestnuts, cashews and peanuts.

• Bean sprouts from mung beans, chickpeas, alfalfa etc. Eat when the sprouts are still short, long before any sign of leaves appear. The shorter the sprouts, the greater the concentration of protein, before it gets used up in the sprouts' rapid growth. (See page 52 for how to sprout your own.)

• Lentils and dried beans (see page 50 for how to prepare and cook these safely).

• Soya products (see opposite).

• Mushrooms (if tolerated), and meat substitutes created from fungi.

• 'Creamy' fruits. These are mostly exotic varieties, but which are increasingly available: custard apple, coconuts, jackfruit, durians (delicious if you can find a source and put up with the smell) and lychees, as well as dates and figs.

• Avocados.

• Tropical vegetables: water chestnuts, drumstick pulp (the insides of a long, tough pod that tastes like asparagus when cooked), palm hearts and yams.

• Ghee (rarified butter), milk and cottage cheese, if dairy products are permitted.

soya

The source of many useful nutrients for strict vegetarians, the soya bean is high in protein and is one of very few non-animal foods to contain all eight essential amino acids. It is also high in vitamins B_1, B_6 and E, and several minerals, including potassium. Therapeutically, soya lowers cholesterol, boosts the immune system and, being high in fibre, eases constipation.

Soya beans are extremely versatile. Unusually for beans, they have a high fat content (mostly polyunsaturated), so as well as being used like any other dried bean, they can be boiled and processed into a creamy constituency to make soya 'milk', 'cream' and even 'yoghurt'. Drained, set and pressed into blocks, soya milk makes bean curd (tofu), which can be cooked in a variety of ways as a stand-in for meat. Tofu has virtually no taste, but absorbs the flavours of spices and well-seasoned sauces. The setting agent used to make tofu also provides calcium. Soy sauce is made from fermented soya beans and a number of additives, including a great deal of salt.

Research into phytochemicals (see page 21) has shown that soya contains phytoestrogens, and so may help with irregular periods, premenstrual syndrome, menopausal hot flushes and post-menopausal problems such as osteoporosis, fatigue and vaginal dryness. It may also help guard against other cancers, including prostate, but because phytoestrogens function like natural oestrogen, there is a question mark over its suitability for young boys. Soya is also one of the more common foods to which susceptible people are allergic.

no meat or fish

Eggs and cheese will still supply first-class proteins (see page 14), but do not over-indulge in them; look to pulses and nuts as sources too. Cheese is high in saturated fat (and blue and rinded soft cheeses contain fungi that you may want to avoid), and too many eggs can cause constipation in some people. Anyone with a high cholesterol count (see page 16) should eat only moderate amounts of both.

Oily fish is a good source of the form of vitamin A called retinol (vital for eyesight and disease resistance). Ensure you get plenty of red, orange and dark green fruit and vegetables instead (these are high in beta-carotene, another form of vitamin A that the body can convert into retinol when it's needed).

Seafood is also where a lot of our vitamin B_{12} (needed for manufacture of blood) comes from, so you will need to rely on eggs, cheese and seaweed.

no meat, fish, eggs or dairy produce

Without these your only source of first-class protein will be soya (see above). Ensure you are getting all the amino acids you need by combining a variety of pulses with potatoes, grains (which includes pasta) and nuts. There is an ever-increasing range of vegetarian products on the market, but check their labels carefully for additives.

To give taste and interest to bases such as tofu (bean curd) and meat substitutes manufactured from fungi, a variety of flavour enhancers and other additives are sometimes used. And if a range is used, each in small quantities, these may not even be listed among the ingredients.

You will need to get your calcium from dark green vegetables, seeds, nuts (especially almonds) and soya milk and tofu that has been enriched with calcium. You must also make sure you are balancing this with enough vitamin D to absorb the calcium (see page 17).

Ward off anaemia with plenty of dark green vegetables and nuts, along with pulses and cereals, to provide you with iron in the absence of meat. Your body will need to use vitamin C to aid absorption of iron from these sources.

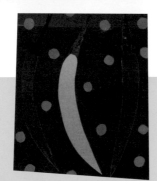

chillies

Hot peppers are used to stimulate appetite in tropical countries, where heat slows digestion and appetite. They boost energy, promote circulation of blood and encourage sweating. Capsaicin, the active ingredient that produces the sensation of heat, is both an irritant and a counter-irritant. Contact with sensitive areas such as the eyes can cause stinging and inflammation, but chilli oil or chilli balm is useful in treating pain, herpes or shingles, rheumatoid arthritis or other forms of inflammation. It helps to thin blood (preventing clotting) and can protect against heart disease, as well as help an overactive or irritated bladder (when in small doses). Green chillies can help to alleviate pain of all sorts (menstrual, headache, arthritic), but as they stimulate acid secretion in the stomach, they should be used in moderation. Another reason for caution is that chillies are generally addictive – the flushing, palpitation, clear head, sweating, salivation and improved moods mimics the kick of drug-induced pleasure which perhaps leaves you wanting to experience it again and again.

Your intake of vitamins B_{12} and D will be minimal. Vitamin D should not be a problem if you see plenty of sunlight; in its absence, seaweed is a useful addition to the diet (it also provides iodine), otherwise you will have to resort to supplements. Without eggs or milk, for B_{12} you will need to look to 'fortified' breakfast cereals and soya products or brewer's yeast (if yeast does not cause problems for you; see pages 44–5).

Vegans who do not take particular care to supplement their restricted diet may suffer from eyesight problems (lack of vitamin A), osteoporosis or arthritis (vitamin D deficiency causes calcium malabsorption), period or hormonal problems (lack of vitamin E) and easy bruising or bleeding gums (vitamin K deficiency).

Apart from nutritional concerns, a strictly vegetarian diet has another shortcoming. Meat and fat stay longer in the stomach than vegetables and take longer to digest, so the feeling of satisfaction lasts longer. Many people, especially those new to vegetarianism, feel hungry much of the time and end up eating a lot of bread and cheese, or sweets.

'heating' and 'cooling' foods

Traditional physicians used to categorise food as 'heating' or 'cooling'. In the East this is still done today. The terms are derived from the need to try to put digestion in terms understandable to the layman. Digestion was thought to be a process similar to cooking, so foods that promoted metabolism, or the conversion of food into energy, were described as 'heating', and those that slowed down metabolism, producing less energy, were known as 'cooling'. Foods can still be classified in this way.

Heating foods require prolonged digestion and generate more heat in the body due to chemical reactions and the increased calorific content. (At the mention of calories, everybody's mind flies to 'calories = weight', but, as calor implies, calories generate energy via heat.) Such foods improve low blood pressure, increase alertness, restore the sexual libido and so on.

Heating foods are recommended to people with a weak constitution, who are prey to frequent colds and coughs, poor circulation, cold hands and feet, a pale colour, thinning hair, poor appetite, a lack of stamina or chronic fatigue. Excess consumption may cause nosebleeds,

heating foods	cooling foods
red meat and game, including duck and goose liver	fish and shellfish
	chicken
cream and butter	milk
eggs	yoghurt and buttermilk
nuts, especially almonds, cashews, pistachios	bananas
bread	oats
wheat	rice
root vegetables	leafy vegetables
cheese, lards and fats	tomatoes
ginger, cloves, turmeric, cardamom, saffron	thyme, parsley, rosemary, caraway, mint
garlic	coriander, cumin
chillies	cinnamon
pineapple	mango
ripe papaya	raw papaya
apples	oranges
honey	potato
saffron	melon and squashes
fenugreek leaves	berry fruits
alcohol	onions
coffee	leeks
sesame seeds	beetroot
sugar	cucumber

haemorrhoids, anxiety, skin complaints and high blood pressure.

Cooling foods, as you would expect, have the opposite effects. They slow down the body's metabolism, digest easily, calm the mind and cool a fevered body. Many summer foods are cooling – fish, cucumber, summer berries – while winter foods like game and nuts are heating. A preponderance of cooling foods in winter will cause mucus discharge, cold symptoms and headaches, so additional heating foods will give the body's energy a boost. Conversely, cooling foods are suited to summer conditions, when too many heating foods will cause

excessive sweating, poor sleep, constipation and general anxiety.

The odd thing is that the English and American diet tends to be cooling, while the Oriental diet tends to be heating. My advice is to make sure you have a good balance of 'heating' and 'cooling' foods in your diet. Eating fruit and vegetables in their proper season is also a sensible guide. Macrobiotic, traditional Chinese, Ayurvedic and other schools of thought all classify foods slightly differently, but, as a rule, foods that give you an energy boost and make you feel warm inside are generally heating; the rest can be considered to be cooling.

chapter 4
from acid to yeast – the troublemakers

There are certain everyday ingredients in our foods that cause particular trouble. With the exception of alcohol, we are inclined to take all the following 'danger foods' for granted – often we have no idea we are eating them, for they can be hidden within what we might consider innocuous meals. These make the rule of moderation and diversity in eating ever more important. There is no need for a total ban on any of these foods, but your body will be hard-pressed to cope with all of them in one day. And if your diet includes all of them all of the time then they become real evils.

acid

In the past, people used to get a condition called anhydric gastritis, due to low acid secretion in their stomachs. They would be prescribed hydrochloric acid to assist the stomach acid. Nowadays, people only ever seem to be hyperhydric, or have high stomach acidity. Reasons for this include increased stress, the appearance of certain bacteria called *Helicobacter pylori* and, tellingly, our increasingly cosmopolitan diet.

The gastric juices that work on the food in our stomachs do so in an acidic medium, but once the pulped food passes into the duodenum, the small intestine, it enters an alkaline environment. Although the stomach can secrete more acid through churning, alkaline secretions (from the gall bladder and elsewhere) are limited, so if the food in your stomach is excessively acid, only portions will be released at a time for the duodenum to work on, the rest being delayed in

tolerance thresholds

Some foods and drinks create particular sensations: the palpitations and sweating from hot chillies, the high of chocolate, the slight dizziness and disinhibition of alcohol. Once experienced it is easy to want to chase after these pleasures again. For some people the 'rush' becomes a stimulant they crave, just as if it were a drug. Even orange juice can do it for some. How 'hooked' any one person gets depends on psychological, even genetic, factors.

But our bodies are remarkable at adapting, so the shock effect wears off as our tolerance to such foods increases. This adaptation is mostly a healthy response, but in some people there remains a need

to achieve the heightened sensation, to cross a threshold that is forever being raised. There comes a point when the body has had enough and starts to rebel. The result can range from stomach ulcers to anxiety attacks and addiction.

With foods and drinks that we consciously ingest we can at least measure our intake. What we cannot calculate are the hidden pollutants – fertilisers, pesticides and chemical preservatives. The body also works hard at adapting to these. But we have no way of knowing how well our body is coping or when and how it might react when its tolerance threshold is reached.

the stomach while supplies of bile and alkaline mucus are replenished. Acidic food retained in the stomach is the cause of much digestive disruption such as indigestion (heartburn), regurgitation, burping, gastritis (which can lead to pernicious anaemia) and gastric ulcers.

A number of substances particularly contribute to stomach acidity. These include citrus fruits (lemons, oranges etc.); vinegar; chutneys and pickles; nuts; very spicy food; fried food; seeds; white wine and champagne; brandy; lager, unless it is neutralised by tonic water; some painkillers and anti-inflammatory drugs; and nicotine.

Eating faster than you should, eating food that is very hot in temperature and drinking alcohol without the buffer of food also increase the stomach's acidity. If excess acid is pushed prematurely through into the duodenum, which suddenly releases large amounts of alkaline mucus (to neutralise the acid and prevent it from burning the lining of the intestine), the acid and alkaline mix will produce a lot of gas. This accumulates in the duodenum, so for people who have a lot of bloating and gas the cause is usually excess acid.

Citric acid is particularly pernicious because we are misled. Many people think citric acid and vitamin C are the same thing. This is not the case. Vitamin C is ascorbic acid, not citric acid. Often the two go together because vitamin C likes an acidic medium, which citric acid helps provide. Many oranges have been specifically cultivated to contain more citric acid to make them taste sharper, hoping customers will see this as representing a higher content of vitamin C, but citric acid is very harmful to the body and does no good at all. As is often the case, there is a balance in nature, and the acidic juice of a citrus fruit is balanced by alkaline pith to neutralise it. However, juicing the fruit removes the pith and you are left with all the citric acid. When choosing a citrus fruit, go for the sweeter varieties: satsumas, tangerines or mandarins, and avoid citrus-based juices.

Regrettably, citric acid is used for other commercial purposes, for example to give an orange flavour to soft drinks, which are then heavily sweetened to override the acid taste. This has become so widespread that I feel I have to include citric acid specifically as one of the evils of nutrition.

Ready-made sauces are also highly acidic because they would otherwise grow mouldy too quickly; acid is an effective preservative. The effect of a highly spiced sauce, such as vindaloo, with added acid is like an 'acid bomb' exploding in your stomach.

In short, for digestion to take place in the duodenum, the medium has to be alkaline. Excess acid will disrupt that, so chew food well, consume acid-producing and overly spicy foods sparingly, and allow very hot food to cool slightly before you begin eating.

caffeine

Caffeine constricts the blood vessels and produces general tension in the muscles. As with so many things, this is good in moderation. But where, perhaps, a single cup of coffee will create a state of relaxed alertness, two or three will make you a little edgy, and more will bring on irritableness and palpitations.

Like alcohol, however, the pleasurable effects of caffeine are potentially addictive. As your body adapts it will take more to reach that relaxed-but-alert state. Because of its cumulative effect one should not drink coffee in excess.

Making a rule for yourself – only one coffee a day, coffee only at the weekends, or whatever – is simple, but you also need to be aware that caffeine isn't only in coffee. Many soft drinks also contain high levels of it, particularly those marketed as energy drinks, and there is also caffeine in chocolate and tea, although in smaller amounts.

Although most of the caffeine has been extracted from coffees and colas labelled caffeine-free, the actual process of extraction and the artificial flavourings added to the 'denatured' product may cause other damage. Little work has been done on this, but my observation has been that decaffeinated drinks cause similar effects – insomnia, digestive problems and irritability – and that avoiding them alleviates most of these symptoms. For more on the alternative to a fix of coffee every morning see below and page 113.

alcohol

The consumption of alcohol is huge and growing. Ninety per cent of people in the West drink alcohol, and between 10 and 20 per cent of them have persistent alcohol-related problems. Excessive alcohol puts huge strains on the health services, creates social problems – from road accidents to releasing pent-up aggression in pubs and clubs – and puts financial and social strain on families. That's why I would term excessive drinking as one of the major evils of modern society. There are regular debates and real concern over the effects of unleashing other drugs on society, but alcohol is the

mint

You can make an infusion from the leaves of this therapeutic herb as a great alternative to a cup of coffee. Unlike caffeine, mint tea is a mild sedative and so can induce sleep at night. Breathing in steam infused with mint or mint oil can help clear a blocked nose. Mint is used as an expectorant in cough mixtures and as an antacid to relieve abdominal cramps and gases. The leaves are delicious when tossed in a salad or stirred into salsas and dressings.

'acceptable' drug. It is also a major source of income for the government, through taxation, so concerns over what it is doing to the health of the population at large is tempered by increasing revenues.

We all know people who drink too much, but we are generally inclined to classify our own alcohol intake – however much it may be – as under control, even if we get drunk from time to time. Excess alcohol is a very individual thing, but there are two points worth remembering: alcohol can be very damaging without your being falling-down-drunk every night, and it changes your perception so that once you have had just a glass or two your ability to judge excess consumption is impaired.

First of all, let us look at how the body reacts to alcohol, both chemically and physically. As soon as alcohol reaches the stomach, part of it gets absorbed directly through the stomach wall, one of the few things the stomach does absorb. If there is a fizz, such as with lager, champagne or with added soda, the absorption is increased because the bubbles mechanically stimulate the stomach lining to absorb more alcohol. Chilled drinks also get absorbed more quickly because the cold briefly contracts the stomach, which then absorbs more quickly as it expands again. An empty stomach will absorb more alcohol because there is no food being processed at the same time.

The absorbed alcohol passes next through the liver, whose main role is detoxification. Alcohol is the only substance that the liver meets that it has to oxidise (turning the alcohol into carbon dioxide and water). If the amount of alcohol is small or slow there is normally no problem, but the liver simply cannot cope with a sudden rush. When this happens, much of it passes through the liver and straight into the bloodstream without being processed.

Once the alcohol is in the bloodstream it joins the regular circulation of the blood, through the heart and round the body, including the brain. The brain's very sensitive cells are heavily protected, first by the cerebral fluid in which it is bathed, and second by a blood–brain barrier that makes it hard for any chemical in the blood to pass through into the brain. Medicines intended to reach the brain have to be very finely tuned to breach this barrier. Alcohol, being a simple molecule, can penetrate it easily. It then causes the well-known symptoms of dizziness, mood enhancement and delirium.

Each time the alcoholised blood flows through the liver a little more is processed, so how long alcohol stays in the system depends on the amount imbibed and the efficiency of the liver. The liver can treat around one unit of alcohol (one small glass of wine or half a pint of beer) an hour, so one night's heavy late-night drinking will still not have been treated by the next morning.

effect on the stomach

This depends on your choice of drink. The basic constituent of alcohol is ethanol, but alcoholic drinks taste very different because of their other ingredients, such as tannin, sugar and flavourings. White wines (including sparkling wines) are acidic and can contribute to all the problems described on pages 40–41. Red wine, in moderation, is an aid to digestion, but beware of the effects of excess tannins and additives to cheap wines. Beer contains too much yeast (see pages 44–5). Spirits are much stronger and can cause ulcers. Fancy liqueurs and cocktails can contain a variety of additives and preservatives.

effect on the liver

The strain that excess alcohol puts on the liver raises the level of toxins in the blood, causing that morning-after hangover. Liver cells that have to process a lot of alcohol over a long period become dehydrated and deprived of oxygen, so they begin to malfunction. Initially fatty deposits make some cells inactive, then if the alcohol intake remains high, fibrous tissue grows to seal them up. This stage, when the liver becomes hard and inactive, is called cirrhosis.

effect on the rest of the body

Alcohol is hygroscopic, that is, it absorbs water, leaving cells dehydrated. When the cells that make

how to drink beer

Beer is gassy. If you sip it, when the chilled beer hits the heat inside your body, the gas will come out instantly in small amounts. But if you gulp it, your stomach is chilled rather than the beer warmed, and the gas will accumulate and rush out later when the temperature is restored. If you drink beer in gulps with pauses in between, the gas is retained in the depths of the stomach and beyond. Four or five pints in a night and the gas accumulation is huge. It disrupts digestion and stretches the walls of the stomach. Aided and abetted by the high calories in beer, this is how 'beer bellies' get made. So, sip your beer and enjoy it in moderation.

blood are deprived of fluid the heart rate goes up and, because they can only function with a certain moisture content, the chemical reactions in the body slow down or stop. After the alcohol is absorbed it releases the water into the urinary system, bypassing the cells which needed it.

Alcohol is also high in calories but with negligible nutritional value. Gaseous drinks such as beer, especially in large volumes, will make you feel full but without providing significant nutrients. If you cut down on your food intake because of this, you are in danger of depriving yourself of vital nutrition. On the other hand, if you eat enough to keep you healthy and take in a lot of 'empty' alcoholic calories you are likely to become overweight.

effect on the mind

The psychological causes and effects of excess alcohol are myriad and very individual. It disrupts sleep patterns; can make people violent, amorous or just plain silly; removes the barrier of inhibitions; creates a delirious state; brings on exultation or deep depression; and creates addictions.

addiction

A tendency towards an addictive dependency on alcohol may be genetically predetermined. A very heavy drinker may suffer the physical withdrawal symptoms from alcohol, but not the psychological ones. Both, however, are in danger of suffering from the same problems by raising their tolerance thresholds to dangerous levels: a lack of concentration, incoherence and slurred speech (even when not drunk). One of the effects of a cirrhotic liver is getting drunk more quickly because of the inability of the liver to extract the alcohol before passing the blood into the bloodstream.

Not every heavy drinker is an addict, but a lot of people don't realise they are addicted until they try to give up. Addictive substances create withdrawal symptoms – one way of testing if a substance is addictive for you is to check the effect its sustained absence has on you. One of the painful realities of any addiction is the withdrawal symptoms, for which the only relief the addict can find is another fix.

sugar

This gives us more than just a pleasing sweet taste. Glucose keeps the brain alert but depresses the appetite, which is why sweet dishes are served at the end of a meal. It is better to pause between the main meal and dessert as the sugar suppresses the digestive process to some degree and you do not want this to happen while the digestion of the rest of the meal is hard at work. For the same reason, the best time to eat fruit is between meals. Try to avoid dessert at night, because it can keep the brain overactive and make sleep difficult.

Extrinsic sugar (that is, sugar that has been extracted from its original source, rather than still being part of – intrinsic to – a fruit or vegetable) comes in many guises, which can make it difficult to keep track of how much you are actually taking in. This is a particular worry in children's diets, as many foods and soft drinks designed to appeal to children are extremely high in various sugars. Often these are listed as separate ingredients on labels, which gives a false impression of the total content. Tooth decay is not the only danger – hyperactivity

is often a result of overdosing on hidden sugars.

Replacing sugar with artificial sweeteners is a bad idea. First, these are made with chemicals, some of which can be very toxic, especially to the liver; only time will tell what the cumulative effects of these will be in the long term. Some are carcinogenic.

Secondly, they fool your taste buds. You may be reducing your sugar intake, but you are not adapting your body to crave sweetness any less.

yeast

Whereas excess alcohol is one of our body's oldest enemies (in the Bible, Noah got famously drunk), yeast is a new one. Quantities of bread in the diet never caused digestive problems unless you had an intolerance to wheat, and people would take brewer's yeast for its B vitamins. But yeast has become a major problem because of the indiscriminate use of antibiotics as medicine and in animal feeds.

The imbalance that antibiotics have caused between fungi and bacteria means that yeast, which for thousands of years has been used in the preparation of bread and alcohol, has now become a problem for many people.

If there is a lot of yeast in the gut and it grows too strong, then it and the body's 'good' bacteria compete for food. A particular problem is *Candida albicans*, a type of fungus which has tentacles (mycelia). To suck out nutrients it drives its tentacles into the duodenum or intestinal walls. Breaching the barrier between the stomach and the intestinal blood vessels like this allows molecules, including toxins, to pass through into the bloodstream. This is commonly known as leaky gut syndrome. These particles are eliminated as mucus in the sinuses and allergic reactions like skin rash. People with a yeast and candida overgrowth also feel very tired.

Another feature of yeast is that it ferments. The spontaneous production of alcohol in the stomach has been known traditionally for centuries. Anyone who has made wine at home knows that the formula is any vegetable or fruit, plus yeast, plus warmth, plus sugar. The stomach, supplied with carbohydrates, yeast and sugar, provides just the right atmosphere in which to brew alcohol. And some of the forms of alcohol it produces are highly toxic, especially to the liver.

The types of alcohol formed in the gut produce excessive lethargy. Have a lunchtime sandwich, swill it down with a sugary drink, and you run the risk that an hour or two later it will begin turning to alcohol. Those who eat yeast products such as pizza, bread or beer, often notice that a little while later they feel heady and very drowsy. This lasts for an hour or two and the fatigue is often overwhelming, but they cannot fathom why.

This 'gut-brewed alcohol' will not show up on a breathalyser, or even a blood test for ethanol (the alcohol found in alcoholic drinks), but drivers and pilots might get a shock if they were tested for other forms of alcohol such as methanol or propinol. Sometimes, perhaps surprisingly, the alcohol level can be so high in the bloodstream that people (including non-drinkers) become delirious, drowsy and are even sick. I wonder if the success rate of organisations helping recovering alcoholics would be higher if they paid more attention to diet to ensure that their apparently abstemious members were not brewing their own alcohol inside?

If you are not well and have problems of gas, lethargy after food, allergies or a skin irritation, try cutting out yeast. People who don't suffer in this way, of course, can eat all the yeast they like. But in my opinion 80 per cent of people these days have gas or digestive problems, and the moment they give up yeast they feel better.

As well as avoiding products high in yeast, there are several other things that affect yeast overgrowth:

• Bile is a natural suppressant of yeast. So anything that reduces bile production or affects the liver, such as contraceptive pills, hormone replacement pills and some drugs, will reduce bile secretion and allow yeast growth.
• Too much acid in your food neutralises bile and so also encourages yeast growth.
• Sugar is a vital ingredient in alcohol, so you should avoid excess sugars (fructose, the form of sugar found in fruit and honey, is fine up to a limit).
• Other fungi, such as mushrooms or cheeses, can cause bloating, gas, allergies or sensitisation if eaten in large quantities.

foods high in yeast

• Bread (including many flat breads such as pitta bread and naan).
• Pizza bases.
• Beers.
• Yeast extract spreads.
• Soy sauce.
• Many canned products.
• Brewer's yeast (often used as a B vitamin supplement).

chapter 5
the healthy kitchen

Both the nutritional benefits and the enjoyment of food are enhanced by careful preparation, which goes right back to the catching of the fish, the rearing of the meat and poultry and the growing of the plants. But there is no point in choosing the freshest and the best, and then treating it badly once you get it home. The more of the preparation you have done yourself the healthier it is likely to be. Bypass the pre-prepared, the canned, the just-heat-and-serve and do it yourself.

shopping

The ideal would be to buy food daily, so that it can be eaten as fresh as possible and little wasted. Unless you can do this, plan your meals so that the most perishable foods get eaten first. In the course of a week, eat fish first, then poultry, then other meat. Among vegetables, leafy ones have the poorest rate of survival, then the flowers (cauliflower, broccoli, artichoke), then the fruits (tomatoes, courgettes, aubergines) and finally the roots (carrots, turnips, potatoes).

Take note of sell-by and best-by dates, and avoid buying 'reduced to clear' items, because they are potentially spoiled.

Avoid buying from sources that suggest a laissez-faire attitude to food: butchers who sell cooked and raw meat side by side (which contravenes hygiene regulations), roadside stalls open to car fumes, shops where the food looks tired or there is food past its sell-by date on the shelves. Champion good-food suppliers, from your local fishmonger to organic 'veg box' services.

Having seen the rise in allergies and food intolerances, and the benefit patients have felt after giving up GM foods, I am convinced that this interference in food's genetic structure has an ill-effect on health. In my opinion, no one with a logical mind will accept GM foods, and it is no wonder that supermarkets and restaurants have been quick to put up signs declaring that their products are free of modified food.

signs of freshness

Fish This is highly perishable. Look for the following indications of freshness: scales that are sparkling, not dried out, flesh that is firm not limp and spongy. There should definitely be no strong fishy smell. If you are buying a whole fish, raise the flap behind the head and look at the gills, the fine fibres through which the fish absorbs oxygen from water. They should be red, not pale or grey. And the eyes should glisten, not look dull and withdrawn into the head.

Meat and poultry Like fish, meat (except game) should not have a strong smell. Texture and colour will vary according to the animal and the cut, but avoid any fresh meat with discoloured patches or dried-up edges. Check frozen meat for freezer burn (pale brown, rough patches). Sometimes antibiotics or chemicals to increase the shelf-life are injected into meat, particularly poultry, which causes brown patches under the skin. If you see this and you have to eat it, soak the meat in a salt and vinegar solution for a couple of hours and then wash it thoroughly before cooking; this will wash out the antibiotics.

Learn to recognise meat with the help of a good butcher, so that you can judge high-quality produce for yourself. Be particularly wary of buying meat from unknown sources, such as market stalls, especially those offering exotic meats at bargain prices.

Eggs There is no mistaking the smell of a bad egg, but there are a number of ways of checking your eggs are fresh. One of the simplest is to hold an egg up to the light: clear and it's good; cloudy and it's not.

Fruit and vegetables Buy organic for freshness. Organic fruit and vegetables have a poor shelf-life and so you can easily tell when they are not fresh. Fruits that have been waxed will retain their moisture content and look good for longer – too long. Potatoes, onions or garlic bulbs that have begun to sprout will have poor nutritional value, because the nutrients have been used in the vegetables' effort to regrow. Leaves that are limp and vegetables that are rubbery rather than crisp and firm have been lying around for too long and will have lost a proportion of their vitamins.

decoding food labels

Labelling on tins, jars, cartons and pre-packed fresh foods can be very informative about the contents, but you need to read the small print.

nutritional information

This will tell you the constituents of the contents: carbohydrates/sugars, protein, fats (divided into saturated and unsaturated), minerals and vitamins. These will usually be listed per 100 g and also, where applicable, per serving. Use the former to compare brands and the latter to tell you how much of each it will be contributing to your diet.

ingredients

These are listed in order of proportion of the total weight (you will be surprised how many begin

seasonal foods

Which tastes better, a strawberry freshly picked in summer or a forced hothouse variety imported in the middle of winter? No contest. Out-of-season strawberries may not do any major harm, but the way they have been grown and the time spent in storage inevitably lowers their food values (and raises the price). We have grown so used to having all foods available all year round that our palates become used to the reduced flavour and texture of much of what we eat. We then exclaim over a truly fresh fruit or vegetable in its prime, forgetting that this is the norm. A healthy, balanced diet should supply all our nutritional needs, but by eating what is effectively substandard goods we may be kidding ourselves that our intake of vital vitamins and minerals is sufficient.

Medieval peasants would survive through the winter on stored food – largely dried beans, root vegetables and some salted meat and fish. In spring and summer, however, these would be supplemented by a variety of greens, including nettles and watercress picked from the wild. In India date palm sap is a popular winter ingredient in many dishes. This sweet sap provides a good

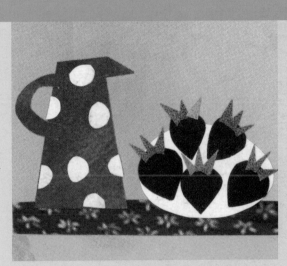

nourishment and is a very powerful diuretic during the months when our bodies tend to be very sluggish.

We are fortunate to have an enormous variety of foods to choose from – not for us the monotonous diet of the medieval peasant or the poor in the Third World. Paying attention to the freshness of our food and enjoying seasonal fruit and vegetables when they are at their optimum quality, however, will bring lasting health benefits.

with 'water'). Look out in particular for:

• **Sugars/sweeteners.** These are each listed separately, which means you can see whether artificial sweeteners have been used, but it may make the sugar element appear less than it is. See page 44 for a list of ways in which these may be described, and use the nutritional information on the label as a gauge to overall sugar content.

• **Vinegar (acetic acid).** Often used as a preservative, to prevent fungal or bacterial growth. Look out for its use in ready-made pasta and cook-in sauces (especially stir-fry).

• **Stabilisers, flavourings, colourings, preservatives.** These are mostly the ingredients that you would never use in home cooking. They may be named or listed by E number. The best advice is: the fewer E numbers the better.

Food manufacturers have to abide by quite strict labelling regulations, but they are also trying to make it sound as attractive as possible. It is a pity to have to be sceptical, but be alert to wording like:

• **-Flavoured.** This means it is made to taste like the flavour (orange, raspberry, etc.), not that orange or raspberry features at all in the ingredients.

• **Low-sugar, sugar-free.** Check the label for sugar alternatives.

• **Meat.** Regulations are becoming stricter on the definition of meat in labelling, but it can cover a lot of unattractive elements such as pulped gristle. Meat substitutes are usually soya-based, and soya is a common allergen (see also page 37).

• **Low-fat, reduced fat.** This means it is lower in fat than the standard variety, not necessarily that it contains little fat.

spices

For centuries, spices were treasured for their therapeutic properties. A belief in their ability to cure the plague, relieve ague and generally ward off all manner of disease gave them almost magical status. As time passed, however, they came to be appreciated more for their taste than their medicinal properties. Rediscover the healing powers of the following spices ...

cardamom

Cardamom is a digestive spice, useful for relieving abdominal cramps, and the oil has antibacterial properties. It also improves circulation, and tea spiced with cardamom boosts energy.

cinnamon

The bark of the cinnamon tree is used to treat diarrhoea, nausea and loss of appetite. It also improves circulation by toning up the heart. Its antibacterial and antifungal properties make it valued as a food preservative and toothpaste.

cloves

A powerful painkiller, clove oil is used to treat toothache, abdominal cramps and externally for muscular or joint pain. Cloves aid digestion and stimulate the secretion of enzymes in the gut.

mustard

Mustard improves circulation, helps to treat colds and stimulates digestive enzymes. It has anti-inflammatory properties and can be used to treat sinuses (as oil drops) and arthritis when used as a rub.

saffron

Saffron boosts the body's energy and immune system, and aids digestion. It can be used as an antibacterial to treat cuts and wounds. Beware of saffron sold as a powder rather than individual stamens as this is often highly adulterated.

turmeric

In Ayurvedic medicine, turmeric (haldi) is highly regarded. It regulates liver function and facilitates bile flow. It acts as an antacid for stomach ulcers and has antibacterial and anti-inflammatory properties.

life in a freezer

Freezing food only delays deterioration, it doesn't postpone it indefinitely, so label everything you freeze clearly with the date. Most meat and vegetables will have a recommended freezer life of 6–12 months, but I think that 3 months is a more sensible limit, with 1 month for:

- Chicken breasts.
- Smoked salmon.
- Ice cream.
- Puddings.
- Fish fingers.
- Burgers and minced meat.

Ensure the temperature in the freezer remains at below –18°C and don't attempt to save and refreeze food after a breakdown or serious power cut.

Foods that shouldn't be frozen at all are:

- Eggs.
- Bread (the yeast spores become very active on thawing, like a rush of growth in spring after the dormancy of winter).

storing and preserving food

There is no doubt that fresh food wins out over preserved. Who can argue against the fact that frozen foods do not 'feel fresh'? Fruit from cold storage houses lose their taste and nutritional value, while pickled or preserved foods lose their freshness.

chilling

Fridges have become essentials in every kitchen. The low temperature and darkness certainly keep food fresh for longer, but it is important to treat it as short-term storage and not to allow things to linger. Warmth and light will hasten spoilage, so avoid keeping fresh food on the work surface or in a warm kitchen cupboard. The exception to this is fruit that you want to ripen more fully.

freezing

Take care when freezing fresh food (see above). Wrap well against freezer burn and freeze as quickly as possible (most freezers have a fast-freeze facility). Don't put too much unfrozen food into the freezer at once or it will raise the temperature inside the freezer. Briefly blanch fruit and vegetables first to avoid their enzymes spoiling them. When buying frozen food, wrap in a cool-bag and get it home and into the freezer as soon as possible; thawed food should not be refrozen.

bottling and canning

Commercially canned and bottled foods use various chemicals (in permissible doses), because manufacturers understandably fear the consequences of a batch of tins or bottles being contaminated by bacteria. It is difficult to know what the long-term effect on our health might be from the regular ingestion of these, which is why I recommend avoiding them.

In theory, bottled foods require no artificial preservatives, so home-made pickles, chutneys, bottled or preserved fruit and vegetables don't receive the same thumbs down. The preparation includes some form of natural preservative, usually salt, vinegar or sugar syrup, and the exclusion of air prevents oxidation.

smoking and drying

Smoking and drying are traditional methods of preservation, especially of meat and fish. These will need to be kept in a dry place if they are not to develop moulds, but they have a good life and retain many of their nutrients. Take account of extra salt when you are rehydrating and cooking, and check labels for preservatives.

kitchen hygiene

Food poisoning from E. coli, salmonella or other contaminants hits the headlines from time to time

and leads to scare stories about unhygienic food. Most problems, however, have their roots in domestic kitchens. Make sure that:
• You separate raw and cooked food, both when storing and preparing.
• Meat is not stored in the fridge above other foods on to which it might drip blood.
• Food does not sit around in a warm room (such as the kitchen). Bugs proliferate quickest at room temperature, so keep hot food hot and, if it is supposed to be left to cool, cover it and put it somewhere it will get cold as quickly as possible (but not the fridge as it will raise the temperature).
• Worktops, especially chopping blocks, are kept scrupulously clean.
• You wash your hands before you handle food, and between touching raw and cooked meat or fish.
• It becomes second nature to children to wash their hands before they eat.
• Pets are kept clear of all food for human consumption, and from kitchen worktops.
• You don't spread infection by sneezing or coughing near food.

food preparation

To maximise the goodness you can obtain from your raw ingredients, you need to know how to prepare them in the right way.

washing beans and grains

All seeds and grains are covered with a powdery substance that has antibacterial and antifungal properties so that the nutritious endosperm of the seed is not attacked. These powdery deposits can cause us flatulence, discomfort and intolerance. If you cook lentils without soaking them first you'll see how much longer the cooking process takes and how much gas they produce inside you later.

Soak lentils and beans for several hours or overnight, refreshing the water a few times, until the water runs clear. Do not soak them for longer than this or they will begin sprouting.

store cupboard staples

Life will be a lot easier if you have to hand the following cooking basics (see illustration opposite):
• A variety of pastas.
• Rice, both long- and short-grain.
• Dried pulses and lentils.
• Couscous.
• Oats (for porridge and crunchy toppings).
• Breakfast cereals.
• Flour.
• Olive oil for cooking and dressings.
• Chutneys and pickles.
• Selection of spices and freeze-dried herbs.
• Salt and pepper.
• Unrefined brown sugar.
• Tea.
• UHT or dried milk (for emergencies).
• Canned fish (in salt water only).
• Honey.

Unless you are shopping every day there are some shorter-lived items it is always useful to keep in stock, from which you can make a meal without resorting to fast food or phoning the nearest takeaway:
• Eggs.
• Yoghurt.
• Butter.
• Cottage cheese.
• Garlic.
• Root ginger.
• Chillies.
• Root vegetables, which last well if stored in a cool, dry place.
• Frozen home-made or good-quality stock (avoid cubes).

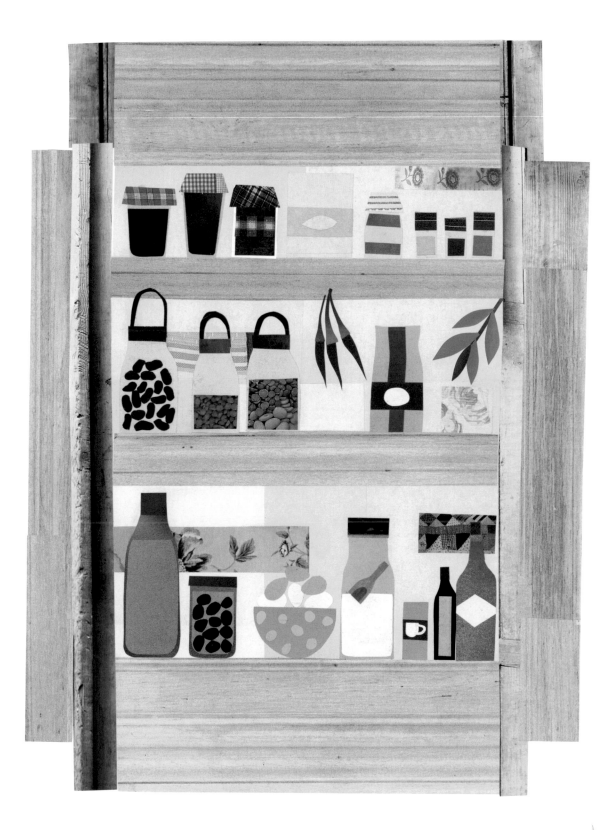

Rice and softer grains like millet or crushed oats do not need prolonged soaking. An hour or even half an hour is long enough. Again, rinse away the powdery deposit. This powder makes rice very sticky, so thorough rinsing will also keep the grains fluffy and separate as they cook.

peeling and cutting

Foods, especially fruit and vegetables, start losing their vitamin content as soon as they are harvested. Peeling and cutting accelerates the degeneration of vitamins A and C, so don't cut up food too soon before cooking. Vitamin C is concentrated just under the surface of fruit and vegetable skins, so either retain the skins and just scrub well, or use a peeler rather than a knife to skim off the thinnest layer of skin.

tenderising

Flesh is firm because the soft fibres of protein are contained within tough sheaths containing collagen. Sustained heat will break up these sheaths, but to reduce cooking time, you can start the process by tenderising meat or fish beforehand. Meat such as steak or escalopes can stand up to being physically hammered to tenderise them, but another method is chemistry. Certain foods, including yoghurt, papaya, lemon juice, vinegar, ginger juice and salt are effective tenderising agents.

Try a marinade of yoghurt and garlic with a little salt and black pepper; red meat will need 2–4 hours, but 30 minutes to an hour is enough for chicken. Pierce meat or fish before cooking to help the flavours penetrate and also to make it easier for heat to reach the centre of the food, further reducing the cooking time. Make diagonal incisions with a sharp knife along the flank of a fish and stab meat with a fork or sharp knife to make deep holes or incisions. Meat from muscular animals, such as game and older organic fowl, can be quite tough and really benefit from a tenderising marinade.

cooking methods

The stomach is perfectly geared up to eat uncooked food like steak tartare, Japanese raw fish, nuts, fruit and vegetables. Cooking, however, makes many foods more palatable and easier to chew and digest. It also introduces new flavours and, in certain cases such as potatoes, renders toxins harmless. (See illustration on page 54.)

how to sprout beans

Bean sprouts are very nutritious and are also easier to digest than unsprouted beans. They are especially high in vitamin C and several of the vitamin B group, and are a good source of protein for vegans.

The hard endosperm of seeds and beans (which after all are really just seeds, too) is a carbohydrates–protein complex. Exposing it to moisture over a period of time breaks the bond and releases the protein which is used for growing, drawing on the carbohydrate for energy. This is what happens when seeds are planted in the soil, and you can do the same in the kitchen – just as you did if you grew mustard and cress on a sponge on the kitchen windowsill when you were young. As well as the familiar bean sprouts (mung beans), you can sprout alfalfa, chickpeas, adzuki and a number of others.

Put a layer of cotton wool on a glass or porcelain dish and moisten it thoroughly with water. Put a handful of washed beans on the bed of cotton wool and wait for the seeds to germinate. Moisten the cotton wool regularly and keep the dish somewhere reasonably warm. The sprouts will grow with or without light, but those grown in light will be green and may be inclined to be bitter.

Most beans will start sprouting within a couple of days and be ready to eat any time over the next two to five days – the time varies according to the size and hardness of the bean. 'Harvest' them when their sprouts are thumb-length or less.

To balance these advantages, remember that:
• Some nutrients are lost or destroyed in heat or are leached into water when boiling.
• Adding too much salt, sugar or spices will completely dominate the actual taste of the food.
• Undercooking can fail to destroy certain bacteria (such as salmonella in raw eggs) that may cause food poisoning.
• Overcooking wastes time and can destroy essential nutrients.

boiling, poaching and steaming

These are the best ways to cook grains, pulses and rice. In fact, it is necessary to ensure that certain pulses, such as red kidney beans, are cooked at boiling point for at least 10 minutes to kill off a harmful enzyme they contain.

Leafy and podded vegetables take little time to cook, so it is easy to overcook them by boiling; they are usually better steamed. When boiling, bring the water up to boiling point first and then add the vegetables, so that they do not spend time leaching their water-soluble vitamins into tepid water.

Dicing hard root vegetables such as carrots, potatoes and turnips increases the surface area. Heat is then absorbed more evenly and the vegetables cook more quickly.

You can retrieve the minerals and some of the vitamins leached out into cooking water by using it as the basis for sauces, soups or stews (although continued boiling will also destroy vitamins).

The stalks of vegetables like cauliflower, broccoli and asparagus take longer to cook than their heads. Separate the heads and add them later, so they don't get overcooked.

The advantage of poaching meat or fish is that you do not need to add any fat. Fish, provided it is not too thick, also steams well – try adding flavourings such as bay and fennel to the water.

Starch, the temperature raiser When boiling a whole cut of meat, such as a piece of boiling bacon or ham hock, plain water will only

cooking fish

Small fish like sardines and trout, and flat fish like plaice or skate are best left whole, and suit being grilled or baked. It is better to cook large, thick fish as fillets or steaks, when pieces can be poached in a sauce or quickly grilled. Fish is a soft, easily spoilt flesh so cooking it in one piece can result in overcooking on the outside before it is done on the inside.

reach 100°C, because that is the temperature boiling water maintains. Here is a tip to increase the temperature of the water and so reduce the cooking time.

Cut up one small potato quite finely and add it to the cooking liquid. The potato will quickly disintegrate, making the liquid starchy and slightly viscous. As the boiling point of starch is much higher, the temperature of the whole dish is raised and the meat will therefore cook more quickly. The temperature can rise as high as 500°C, so watch out that you don't get burnt. If it is not too salty, the cooking liquor can form the basis of an accompanying sauce.

stewing

Casseroling in the oven uses a lower, indirect heat. Food will take longer to cook but there is little danger of it burning or cooking unevenly. Water-soluble vitamins will pass into the cooking liquid, but will not be entirely lost because the juices or sauce will be eaten as part of the meal. Slow cooking tenderises tough meat such as game, which also benefits from being marinaded in a tenderiser (see opposite).

baking

Oven cooking without fats or oils is a good option for many types of food, as the indirect heat means there is a more even distribution of temperature, and no loss of water-soluble vitamins.

As well as baking potatoes in their skins you can give sweet potatoes, onions and garlic the

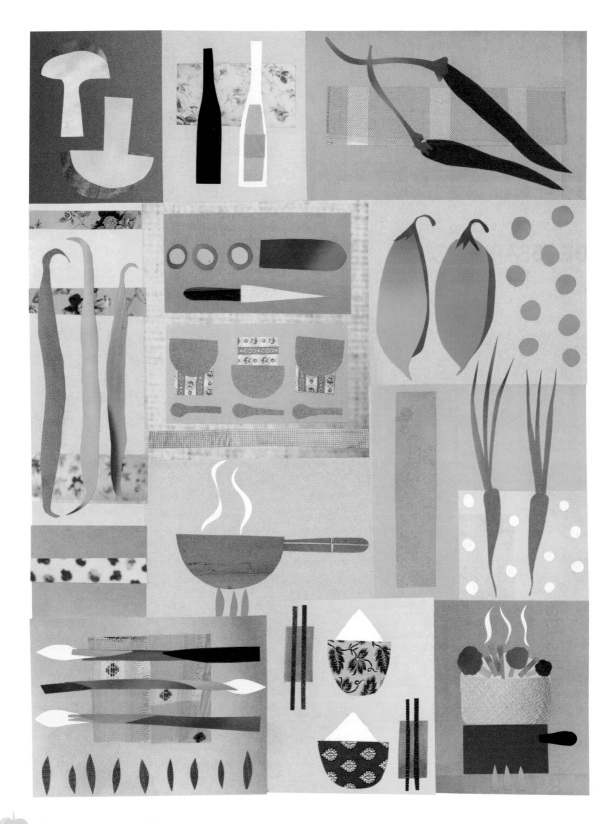

same treatment (bake a whole head of garlic until it is soft and its flesh will become purée-like and lose all sharpness – just squeeze it from the clove skins). Apples, peaches and plums also bake well.

Baking also suits composite dishes such as savoury crumbles and pasta bakes, and baked marrow with a well-flavoured minced meat or rice and vegetable stuffing is an under-rated classic dish.

roasting, grilling and barbecuing

As ways of cooking meat, these have the advantage of forcing fat from the meat (to collect in a tray below). Because of the high temperatures involved, it is necessary to be wary of two things: the meat becoming tough from exposure to high temperatures, and burning the food (charred meat is tasty but there is a worry about carcinogens).

Don't limit your roasting or barbecuing to meat and fish – experiment with root vegetables, tomatoes and corn on the cob.

stir-frying

The very high temperatures used to stir-fry mean that food is cooked very quickly. If you are going to fry, this is the way to do it.

Use a minimal amount of oil and plan the order in which you cook the ingredients. Begin with the items that take longest to cook and finish with those that need least cooking. For example, in a vegetable stir-fry, carrots should be put in first, followed by peas, courgettes, aubergines and finally cabbage or pak choi. Stir-fry mixes sold in supermarkets are convenient, but never work very well as some vegetables end up overcooked.

microwaving

In microwave cooking, the food molecules are broken up and are made to vibrate at a certain frequency, generating heat. This is what happens in conventional cooking, but at a lower frequency, so it doesn't interfere with the food molecules so violently. You may have noticed that food heated up in the microwave gets cold very quickly.

To set against this, the speed of heating and lack of water means that the loss of water-soluble vitamins is much less. However, microwaves are not so good for anything fat-based, such as meat or combinations of foods.

pressure cooking

Perhaps because of the advent of microwaves and horror stories about meals exploding all over kitchen ceilings, pressure cookers are no longer the must-have pieces of equipment they once were. A modern pressure cooker, however, can be a real boon to cooking healthily in a hurry, particularly for stocks, rice and casseroles. The food is, in effect, steamed, but the pressure element reduces cooking time by about half. The shorter cooking time means more nutrients are retained, and not so many are lost in cooking water. Never pressure-cook pulses and lentils in a hurry. Not only do they not taste very good but they will produce a lot of gas and indigestion.

olives

The Prophet Mohammed said that the olive and its oil are the best medicinal products nature has provided. It is a very versatile oil to cook with: use it in stir-fries, salad dressings, bakes, stews and sauces. Olives contain zinc, mono-unsaturated fats and essential oils that cut cholesterol, improve blood pressure (when low), stimulate energy and strengthen the immune system. The oil is also used for the treatment of arthritis, both externally and internally.

chapter 6
resting your digestive system

We all recognise that we need to rest every night, and look forward to giving our minds and bodies a break with holidays. Our digestive systems, which keep going every day of the year, also benefit from a rest. Sometimes our bodies tell us to give our digestion a break. We all go through phases of losing our appetite, perhaps because we have overeaten the night before or don't feel well. A sick baby or a sick dog will not eat, and, often, nor do we. This is because the body is taking time off to deal with the sickness, concentrating our energy elsewhere than on the digestive system.

fasting for health

There is no doubt that fasting from time to time does the body a lot of good. Here are some benefits of fasting:

• It gives the digestive system a rest and an opportunity to carry out maintenance work, from healing ulcers and regenerating damaged tissues or lining to simply resting the muscles that help to churn the food.

• It helps the liver. The liver has to detoxify everything that is absorbed from the intestines before letting it into the main bloodstream. During fasting one avoids fats, alcohol and heavy meals – all the things that make the liver have to work the hardest.

• You lose weight.

• It builds up willpower and the desire to help the body to heal itself.

• It de-stresses the body. Quality of sleep improves, and our mood lightens as internal body disturbances (aches and pains, lethargy, rumbling in the abdomen, discomfort from the intestines, muscle tension and so on) do not distract the mind subconsciously.

• It enhances the innate healing power to combat diseases.

preparing for a fast

Don't think you need to eat as much as possible the day before to carry you through. This is quite wrong! Just as you should introduce your body to a vigorous physical work-out by starting with some warm-up exercises, you should 'wind down' your digestion the evening before a fast. Make dinner something light and easy to digest, like soup and salad.

Make sure that you have a good supply of water (flavoured if you prefer), fasting tea (see opposite) and, if you need them, fruits. This should be a quietly enjoyable time, so plan how you will spend your day or days – have books and music to hand, indulge in some fragrant bath oils or book yourself a massage.

Our desire for food is stimulated by sights and smells, so avoid being where food is. Walk down any high street and you will be assaulted by advertisements for food and the aroma of coffee, so think ahead to avoid these temptations. Empty the fridge if necessary.

Like your last meal, the first meal after your fast should be easily digested, to reintroduce your body to food. Plan ahead, rather than rush out to the nearest takeaway and undo all the good that your abstinence has done.

weekly one-day fast

This gives your digestive system a regular rest one day a week. Choose the same day each week – I prefer Monday as an antidote to socialising and indulging over the weekend. Try not to do anything strenuous or stressful on this day. It will help the mind to relax too.

Most important is to keep up your water intake during the day. Aim to drink at least 1½, preferably 2 and up to 3 litres of water. Alternate plain water with a few cups of fasting tea (make your own, or you can buy my own brand in sachets, see page 220), which is highly recommended to control appetite and promote detoxification.

If your moods really fluctuate when you fast, and there is a risk you might lose control if you have to deal with other people, fruit will help. Three or four portions will provide you with enough glucose but your liver will not object – fruit is easily digested. Eat a serving of fruit in the morning and then two or three times during the day, as you need it. This will see you through even manual work. Melons, grapes, bananas, apples or pears are all good, but avoid citrus fruit. Fresh vegetable juices are another good buffer – try carrot, celery, mint, beetroot or cucumber, either on their own or in combinations.

If you are unused to fasting, if your schedule is tough and you have an uncontrollable desire to eat something, or you feel light-headed or very weak, then make up a vegetable soup (see below) to be eaten at lunch- and dinner time.

When you first do this type of weekly fast your body will ache, and you will get headaches, bad moods, slightly loose stools and extreme fatigue. This is primarily because of the release of toxins and withdrawal symptoms. Drinking sufficient water is important. If somebody can give you a massage in the neck and spine area, most of these symptoms will go away as you relax. A couple of warm showers or an aromatic bath at the end of the day are also great relaxants. This will eliminate muscle ache and improve general circulation (the heat makes the heart race and after the bath you sweat more). As time goes by, these symptoms will vanish and you'll get used to it. Fasting then will be a pleasure.

Break your fast the next morning with porridge or cottage cheese, followed by tea and honey.

bi-annual three-day fast

Every six months or so, treat your body to a three-day fast. You could time these to fall just after periods of over-indulgence, such as Christmas or summer holidays.

Use the three days also to calm your nervous system. Plan to do positive but quiet activities, like reading, listening to pleasant music and swimming. Talk as little as possible. Best of all, take a get-away-from-it-all break. This will refresh the mind as well as the body. Then you will feel on top of the world and not get tired, contrary to what many people say about fasting. This is a misconception of Western culture. In the East people grow up with

vegetable soup

Boil a selection of vegetables – cabbage, carrots, broccoli, peas, courgettes, onions, leeks – in 1½ litres of water for about an hour, until they are overcooked. Blend the mixture to make a thick soup.

fasting tea

Boil 2 cinnamon sticks, 6 cloves, 1 tbsp aniseed and 2 tbsp dried cranberries (optional) in about 1½ litres of water for 5 minutes and leave to infuse. Drink one glass of this infusion with ½ tsp of honey five times a day.

this sort of practice, and deeply religious people know it works and that this is the right way round.

Unless your time is very much your own, a long weekend, Friday to Sunday, makes a convenient time-span. Here's how to do it:

The evening before

Have vegetable soup or vegetables, rice or pasta, or salad and soup.

Day 1

Fasting tea and water. You can work on this day.

fennel

The aromatic oils in fennel seeds control bloating in the abdomen, regulate digestion, and act as an antispasmodic, relieving intestinal and uterine colics. Menstrual cramps are treated with fennel, which also improves breast milk production and helps to control uterine discharge (leucorrhoea and after labour). An infusion of fennel helps sore throats and helps to clear phlegm in catarrh and bronchitis. It can also be used as an eye wash to soothe the itchiness of hayfever or conjunctivitis. Fennel controls appetite and so is a common ingredient in fasting teas.

Day 2

Fasting tea and water. No work should be done on this day. Sleep as much as possible. Keep activity low-key but don't let yourself get bored. Listen to music, read, play chess with someone who is not very good at it, whatever amuses you. Massage and steam/sauna/hot bath (see illustration opposite) are essential as the body will feel tired. (It is a shame that massage is used so little, yet much of the benefit of massage is gained through the healing properties of the hands of the masseur.)

Every day you fast you are taking one step towards self-discipline, willpower and listening to your body.

Day 3

Fasting tea and water all day.
Break your fast at dinner with some vegetable soup (see page 57).

Day 4

Breakfast: porridge, fruit and tea.
Lunch: raw salad (carrots, cucumber, lettuce), vegetable soup and steamed vegetables.
Dinner: vegetable soup, and pasta with vegetables or steamed rice with stir-fried vegetables.

This fast will really make you savour food anew. Eat slowly and you will realise how tasty food can be as your taste buds and sense of smell will be accentuated.

the fasting therapy phenomenon

During the Second World War, Professor Yuri Sergeivitch Nikolaev was working in a psychiatric hospital in the USSR where there was an acute shortage of food. He gave patients water and a weak solution of cranberries and honey. Many got better. That was the beginning of his research, and he established the Soviet School of Medical Fasting.

After Nikolaev successfully treated Kosygin's daughter for psychological problems, the former

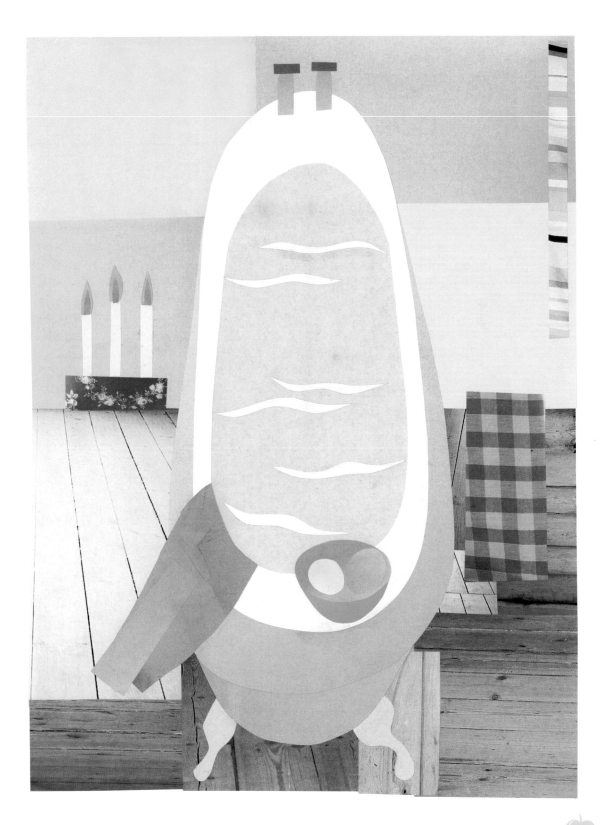

Soviet premier ordered further research into fasting therapy. It was introduced in the treatment of schizophrenia, as an alternative to electric and insulin shock treatments. From the beginning, patients slept better and were considerably calmer during the fasting period. Many became creative, their desires to paint, write and play music adding to the healing process. They showed overall improvement in memory, concentration and libido.

Professor Nikolaev's research proved that his therapy also worked for many physical ailments, such as osteoarthritis, eczema, irritable bowels, allergies, obesity, liver disease, migraine and bronchial asthma. Fasting resulted in a most amazing improvement in liver function in people affected by alcohol or drug-related conditions, even viral liver problems (hepatitis). The gut lining, after secreting grey mucus in the initial period of fasting, turned pink and erosions or ulcers healed.

There is a phenomenon that puzzles both patients and therapists, including naturopaths, homeopaths and acupuncturists, who use self-healing. Shortly before being cured the body goes through a healing crisis, in which all the symptoms flare up. Patients taking homeopathic remedies often panic, as symptoms such as eczema, mouth ulcers, joint pains, nightmares or migraine get worse. Then they disappear. Many believe that everything 'comes out' of the body at this point, but no one really knows why this happens.

This phenomenon also occurs in fasting therapy if correctly conducted. For the first three days the patient feels very tired, has hunger pangs, is agitated and dreams about food. There then follows a feeling of well-being. The body feels lighter and some of the symptoms of the diseases begin to ease. Suddenly, between the seventh and ninth day of fasting, the healing crisis hits. Professor Nikolaev controlled it with intravenous fluids, enemas, gentle massages, steam baths or saunas and music therapy. Then, almost miraculously, all symptoms disappear and the patient feels well again. From then until the end of fasting (15–20

days) the patient continues to improve. Minor crises might follow, but they are not so uncomfortable.

Such procedures are today practised widely in health farms, but that is how modern fasting therapy began.

At this point I must warn most strongly against attempting a long fast of this nature other than under strict medical supervision.

A footnote: when I was studying clinical surgery in Moscow, I spent time on a ward for vascular surgery. Almost everyone suffering from deep vein thrombosis was treated with fasting therapy. We now know that during fasting, an enzyme, urokinase, is secreted in abundance in the blood. This enzyme and others break down fat to release energy, but before doing so they dissolve recent or fresh blood clots in veins. In the days before bypass surgery, this treatment helped to remove plaque from coronary arteries and restore blood flow to the heart.

can anyone fast?

In some traditions where religious fasts are the norm, children as young as ten fast without problems. In general, however, my view is that fasting before adulthood needs to be handled very carefully. It can be introduced under supervision from about the age of fifteen, but the desire to lose weight, a tendency to anorexia and peer pressure is so high that suggesting fasting to teenagers should only be done with great caution. Fasting together as a family can help. Even then, a total fast is not recommended.

It is also not advisable to fast during menstrual periods, and fasting is not recommended for pregnant women, or women trying to conceive. However, a 'vegetarian day' or a 'cleansing day' perhaps once a month, limiting your diet to fruit, vegetables, eggs and fish, is a safe way of giving your digestion a bit of a holiday. Check with your doctor or gynaecologist before embarking on a new regime.

After you reach the age of 40 it is increasingly sensible to fast, as your system copes less well with being put under constant strain. An elderly person may not be able to undergo a full fast unless used to doing so, but giving the digestion a periodic rest from meat, fat, carbohydrates such as cakes and chocolate, and alcohol, is important for your well-being. A sensible compromise is to undertake a semi-fast once a week or once a fortnight, with fruit and vegetables (including salad) and, of course, plenty of water and fasting tea. Again, discuss what is best with a qualified professional, especially if you are suffering from any chronic complaints such as osteoporosis, extreme low blood pressure or arrhythmia.

religious fasting

The principle of abstinence – forgoing not only greed but lust, anger and other strong emotions – was traditionally seen as a route to health and bodily control and to achieving spiritual awareness. It has long been incorporated into religious practices, possibly in recognition of the healing power and spiritual uplift associated with fasting. Many religions promote fasting as a method of self-purification and sacrifice, including Christian Lent, Jewish Yom Kippur, the nine-day Hindu fast of Navatra, and the Islamic month of fasting, Ramadan. Often these periods are followed by a significant festival.

It is unfortunate when the letter, rather than the spirit, of the fast is followed. When this happens, observing Lent becomes reduced to giving up chocolate or, during Ramadan, people stay awake all night, eating past midnight and then sleeping off their excesses during the daylight hours. The entire purpose of the fast is lost. Balance a daytime fast during Ramadan with fruit, soups and plenty of water after sundown and the body would then certainly be healing itself.

Whether you are religious or not, these periodic semi-fasts have much to commend them. I strongly recommend an extended Lent, starting shortly after the New Year (following the overeating and drinking over the Christmas period) and lasting until Easter Sunday. I normally advise people to refrain from smoking and drinking alcohol or coffee during this period, and to eat one main meal a day consisting of light, easily digestible foods like grilled fish and vegetables. For breakfast eat fruit and drink herbal tea and for lunch or dinner a vegetable soup and raw salad. It is better to avoid puddings and excessively oily or buttery food. It is a wonderful way of shedding weight and cleansing oneself. As with a shorter fast, reintroduce your body slowly to heavier foods.

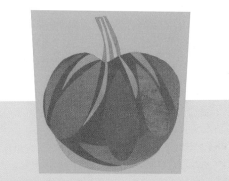

pumpkin

Squashes like pumpkin were one of the first domesticated plant species. Pumpkin is a diuretic, used to treat kidney problems, constipation, heat stroke, irritable bladder and prostate problems. The presence of zinc helps to boost the immune system. Marinated in a syrup, pumpkin is good for regulating the bowels and controlling stomach acid in gastritis or ulcers. The tasteless white pumpkin known in India as petha is used there to cleanse the gastro-intestinal tract during fasting – its juice is recommended during a prolonged fast (7–10 days) to neutralise the enzymes and detoxify the body.

chapter 7
regimen therapy

Hippocrates postulated that every one of us possesses an innate healing power or sanogenetic force that not only helps us to overcome disease but also maintains us in good health. In order to activate this healing power, we have to carry out a simple regimen of diet, exercise and massage and to practise moderation. Based on these principles, I formulated my Regimen Therapy. This combines the removal of physical and mental stress (through yoga, see illustration opposite) to generate well-being, optimum nutrition (through regulating the digestive system) and improvement of circulation (through massage).

It is common sense that if we eat well, exercise regularly, manage our stress, improve our circulation, rest and learn to listen to our body's requirements, we are bound to be healthier. A traditional medical practitioner in India will almost invariably start a prescription with *perhez* – a diet and lifestyle regimen. A list of don'ts (relating to habits such as smoking, bathing, sleeping and sex as well as to diet) would be highlighted before the positive recommendations.

yoga

An ancient Indian art of health management, yoga can help to overcome both physical and emotional stress. Through specific movements it moves joints, stretches muscles and tendons, improves general blood circulation, massages internal organs, improves blood flow to the brain and various parts of the body, and alleviates fatigue and sluggishness. With the help of special breathing techniques (known as *pranayama*), yoga stills the mind, restores calmness and improves the functioning of the brain and the rest of the body. Controlled breathing is meditative and builds willpower. A few simple yoga exercises each morning before breakfast are an excellent start to the day, and relaxing poses are recommended at the end of the working day to relieve stress and clear the mind.

complete breath
ujjayi pranayama

This helps increase your lung capacity, relieve tension in your upper spine and open out the mid-chest, decongesting the area.

1 Stand or sit cross-legged on the floor. First, breathe out completely. Then, when you inhale, let your diaphragm relax by letting go of the area below the ribcage. Fill up your lungs slowly and steadily by expanding your chest up and out. Visualise every part of your lungs filling up with air.

2 Next, exhale slowly. Try to make your out-breath longer than your in-breath, but make sure that you are comfortable. Don't pull in your abdomen – let it relax by itself, so that your lungs are passive as they empty. Continue for 10 minutes, keeping the same position and rhythm of breath.

3 When you can perform Steps 1 and 2 without straining, try to hold your breath to achieve a ratio between inhalation, holding and exhalation of 1:1:2. Repeat for 20 such breaths, then lie down and relax in the Corpse Pose (see page 68).

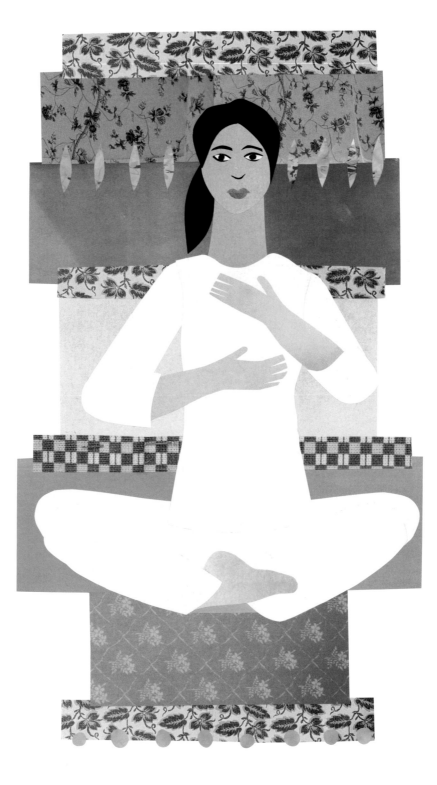

diet

The 'five evils' in the European diet, which time and again are at the root of health problems, are: acid (especially citric), alcohol, caffeine, sugar and yeast. How and why these create such problems are explained in Chapter 4. To these can be added salt and spices in excess, and too much oil and fat. Diets and food preferences vary around the globe, but food is now truly international, so we also need to be wary of things like too much creamy coconut milk and ghee, MSG, fermented soy sauce, smoked and cured meats, and exotic delicacies such as '100-year-old' eggs and half-rotted meat.

Use common sense and logic to determine what is good for your body and what is not. If digestion is not impaired by food and drinks, then the body absorbs what is essential from food and eliminates the waste. Anything that results in indigestion, gas, abdominal cramp, metabolic disorders (gout, diabetes), constipation or signs of food intolerance (skin rash, headaches, chronic fatigue, diarrhoea) is to be avoided as much as possible. You should also try to steer clear of additives and synthetic versions of food or beverages, such as substitute cream, butter, sugar or coffee.

Another important thing to remember is that mixing foods shocks the body and puts tremendous strain on the digestive system. A full multi-course dinner, for example, might easily consist of wine, nuts, canapés, creamy soup, meat, sauces, salads and vegetables, potatoes or rice, bread, butter, dessert, coffee, liqueurs, after-dinner mints and fizzy water all in one meal. This complicated mix requires the body to produce different enzymes and separate the foods so that they can be digested and absorbed – a very strenuous procedure! The simpler the diet the better it is for the body. That is why the diet I prescribe in my Regimen Therapy is so easy to follow yet so beneficial.

This dietary guidance is not about never touching any of the 'bad' foods and drinks. Once in a while (perhaps once a month) you can let yourself go and do all the wrong things in moderation. Just be prepared to skip the next couple of meals or simply eat fruit and drink plain water. This will give the body time to rectify the damage. It would have by then restored the energy, synthesised the overspent enzymes and, most of all, rested the liver from overwork. As an overall guide, my advice is to restrict yourself to one or two 'evils' at a time in a period of 24 hours, and then abstain. Moderation and balance is everything. It is when you consume all the wrong items of food and drink all the time that the body gets confused and overloaded.

More practical guidance on how to incorporate these recommendations into your life are found in Part Two. Here, however, is a summary – an invaluable guide to the management of your diet, whatever your state of health.

10 guidelines to a healthy lifestyle

- Avoid smoking and drinking alcohol.
- Eat organic food, especially when you have meat and poultry.
- Avoid canned and preserved food.
- Avoid yeast products; fried, fatty or oily food; citrus fruits (except tangerines, clementines or oranges that have not been tampered with genetically); cheese; mushrooms; coffee; sodas; energy drinks; excess salt; and refined sugar.
- Balance your intake of fruit and vegetables with sufficient protein. Try to maintain roughly a 60:15:25 proportion of carbohydrates, proteins and fats. If you are vegetarian, you should eat tofu, cottage cheese, nuts and sometimes protein supplements.
- Drink carrot, celery, apple and ginger juice.
- Drink plenty of water, about 2–2½ litres a day.
- Sleep early and rest whenever possible. Do not take your body for granted. Give it plenty of rest. An afternoon nap or siesta is very beneficial.
- Dinner should be light and eaten early.
- Chew well and eat slowly.

healing massage

Have your partner lie face down on the bed or on a few layers of towels laid on the floor. Put a pillow under his or her chest, with the neck at the edge and the head just beyond it.

1 Start by rubbing some massage oil between your hands to warm it up. You can use Dr Ali's Lifestyle Oil (see page 220) or any other oil you like.

2 Grip the shoulders with your hands and, using your thumbs and fingers, squeeze them gently and release. Use your thumbs to rub deep into the shoulder muscles. Some areas will feel 'knotted' and might even be sore. The more you press and release, the better these areas will feel.

3 Grasp the neck with your thumb on one side and your four fingers on the other. Rub the stringy or tight muscles, starting at the top of the neck and working down to the shoulder area. Start with gentle pressure and increase as you go along. Your thumb and fingers should massage the base of the occiput where muscles of the neck are attached. This is often a sore area. Massage and release the tension.

4 Using the balls of your hands, press along the muscles on either side of the spine (about 3–4 cm from the central line or bony part of the spine). Massage up and down. Using the same technique, press deep into the buttocks and use a rotational movement.

5 Move on to the legs. Squeeze the calves between your thumb and fingers and massage downwards. Use your thumb to massage the soles and heels of the feet.

6 Massage the jaw muscles with your thumb. These can get very sore, especially during periods of tension.

7 Finally, massage the scalp with your fingers and thumb.

massage

Among the many benefits of massage are that it:
• Improves the circulation of blood.
• Removes lactic acid from muscles (which is what creates aches and pains).
• Helps to repair the wear and tear in tendons, muscles, ligaments, joints and other tissues.
• Creates a 'feel good' factor that relieves stress and aids healing.

The neck and shoulder massage (see above) that I so often recommend has its own therapeutic benefit. Nature has created two separate circulatory systems for the conscious and subconscious brain. While the conscious brain analyses, makes decisions, thinks and makes voluntary movements, the subconscious brain controls healing, well-being, bodily functions (appetite, hormone regulation, breathing, body temperature control, energy control, posture, heartbeat, sleep etc.) and emotions. A pair of blood vessels, called the vertebral arteries, hidden deep within a canal in the top part of the spine, feed the subconscious part of the brain. Massage of the neck and shoulders helps to reduce tension in the muscles, improving blood supply to the subconscious brain through the vertebral arteries. It is amazing how well one feels immediately after such a massage.

The best time to give or receive a massage is when you are relaxed and not in a hurry. If you have a partner, bedtime is a good opportunity to give each other a soothing, therapeutic massage. The sequence detailed above is designed to take about 15 minutes, and will bring about total relaxation.

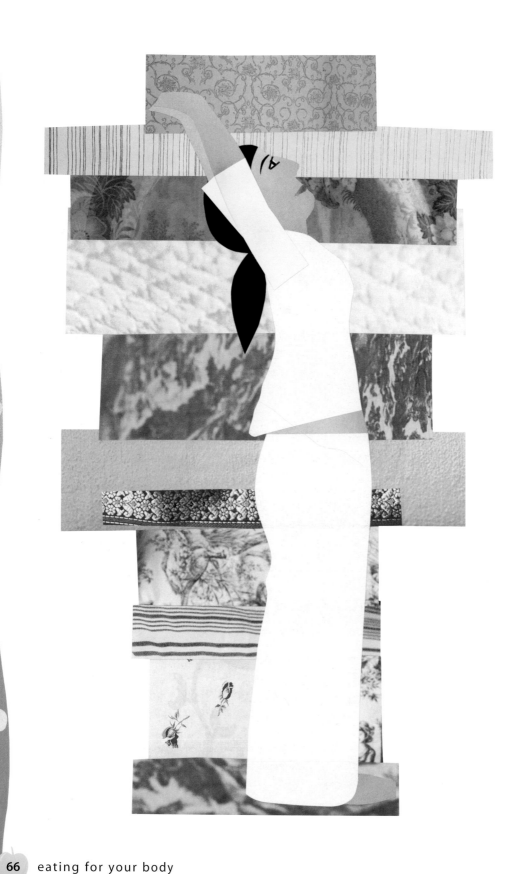

salute to the sun
surya namaskar

Ideally perform this in the morning as it will prepare you for the day ahead. Work through this graceful series of 12 postures slowly, coordinating your breathing with each movement. Use Complete Breath (*Ujjayi Pranayama*) breathing (see page 62) while you are doing this The aim is to reduce the number of breaths required to complete the cycle. For an aerobic workout, repeat for 20 minutes.

1 Stand either with your feet together or hip-width apart if you find it easier. Keep your palms together in front of your chest. Distribute your weight evenly. Take a few slow, deep breaths, keeping your neck straight and your shoulders down. Do not arch your mid-spine, but tuck your abdomen in towards your spine.

2 Inhale deeply, relax the area below the ribcage and expand your ribs outwards and forwards. Lift up your arms and stretch back, pushing your hips forwards but keeping your legs straight (see illustration). Look up. If you have a weak, painful neck, look straight ahead and just stretch up your arms.

3 Breathe out slowly and bend forwards, pulling your arms in front of you before reaching down to place your palms on the floor. Your hands should stay in this position for the rest of the sequence. Lower your head towards your shins, relaxing your neck. If you can, straighten your legs; otherwise bend your knees a little. If your wrists are painful, place your knuckles on the floor.

4 Breathe in and take your left leg back, resting the knee on the floor, with your toes curled under. Stretch your right knee forward while keeping your heel on the floor. Straighten your upper back and neck.

5 Hold your breath and take your right foot back to join the left one. Support your weight on your hands and toes. Keep your spine in line with your head and look at the space in-between your hands.

6 Breathe out and lower your knees towards the floor by bending your arms. If your arms can't hold your weight, then lower your knees to the floor first. Now lower your chest and forehead to the ground without dropping your hips.

7 Breathe in and lower your hips to the floor. Point your toes and then stretch back. Press your shoulders down (you may need to bend your elbows), keep your upper back straight, push your chest forwards and look up.

8 Breathe out, curl your toes under again and lift your hips to form an upside-down 'V'. Stretch your heels down to touch the floor and relax your head. Stretch out your arms, keeping your spine straight.

9 Breathe in and put your left foot forwards in-between your hands. Rest your right knee on the ground and straighten your neck, as in Step 4.

10 Breathe out, bring your right foot forwards next to the left one, straighten your legs and bend forwards, as in Step 3. Try to move from the hips and not the upper back.

11 Breathe in, stretch your arms out in front of you and then lift your arms up and stretch back, as in Step 2.

12 Breathe out, then put your arms into the prayer position. Stand up straight and tall, with your weight distributed evenly. This is one cycle. Repeat 2 cycles to start off with, building up gradually to 12 cycles

corpse pose
shavasana

Although this sounds simple, it is in fact the hardest posture to achieve because it's difficult to let your muscles relax as if you were in a deep sleep while remaining conscious. Steps 2–4 gently stretch the back and sides of the neck and the shoulders, which helps to relax the whole body.

1   Lie down on your back with your feet apart and your legs relaxing outwards; keep your arms a little away from your trunk, palms facing up. Take a deep breath in and lower your chin to stretch the back of your neck away from your shoulders. Breathe out slowly then release the neck and shoulders, allowing them to 'sink' towards the floor. Relax your facial muscles. Your abdomen should rise on inhaling and fall on exhaling.

2   Take another deep breath in, lift your arms up and stretch them out on the ground behind your head. Flex your toes to stretch the back of your legs. Breathe out slowly and relax your arms, feet, legs and neck. Return to normal breathing and slowly lower your arms to your sides again.

3   Take a deep breath in and press your shoulders down away from your neck. Stretch your fingers out and point to your toes with your out-stretched arms. Breathe out slowly and relax again. Return to normal breathing.

4   Breathe in and turn your head to the right so that your right ear is touching the floor. Keep your left shoulder pressed down to the floor. Breathe out and keep this stretch. Then return to normal breathing. Relax the left side of your neck and shoulders. Stay like this for 2–3 minutes, relaxing your facial muscles, particularly the jaw, by taking your tongue away from the roof of your mouth. Repeat on the other side.

5   Lie still and let your mind's eye wander over your body, starting with your toes. Keep your breathing below the ribcage: it should be rhythmic, smooth and light without any constrictions. Relax your muscles completely. Try to let the base of the skull sink deeper and deeper towards the floor. Then check your breathing again. Stay in this posture for 20 minutes.

6   Slowly turn to the right with your right hand under your head. Relax, then slowly roll over and repeat on the left. Turn to the right again to stand up slowly.

blessed posture
bhadrasana

This is very beneficial as it gently opens up the lungs and stretches the neck and vertebral column. Gaze at the tip of your nose, which will help you to concentrate and be calm.

1   Sit on your heels and bring your feet together under your buttocks. Take hold of your right toe with your right hand, and your left toe with your left hand.

2   Lower your chin to your sternum and gaze at the tip of your nose for 10 to 12 breaths. Make sure your breath is slow and even and relaxed. Release the pose and put your left hand into your lap, with your palm facing upwards.

3   Place your thumb on your right nostril to close it and breathe deeply through your left nostril. Then close your left nostril and breathe out through your right nostril. Do the same cycle for the other nostril and repeat both five times.

yoga sleep

The basic principle of yoga sleep is to do the exact opposite from what you have been doing. Where muscles have been contracting, they should now expand and relax. If there has been a deficiency of blood flow, you allow fresh blood to circulate. Yoga sleep is incredibly refreshing and takes just 10 minutes – get into the habit of doing it regularly after lunch and you will really notice the benefit.

Yoga sleep is best practised lying flat on a carpet. But if this is impractical, try to recline in a chair with a headrest, which will support your neck. You can either learn the sequence below and repeat it to yourself mentally, or record it on to a tape.

1 Close your eyes and focus on your neck muscles. They are very tight. Imagine them relaxing; picture a lot of blood rushing into them as they relax. Concentrate on the nape of your neck – you can probably feel the tension in your neck muscles pulling all the ligaments attached to your skull. Let them relax. From one ear lobe to the other, the entire band of ligaments is relaxing. You can feel the tautness going away.

2 Move on to the area lower down your neck. Feel the muscles relaxing. They are dilating and expanding. Go down deeper into the upper chest area. These muscles are attached to the bones in the upper body. Let these ligaments relax. Imagine that blood is flowing in. Imagine that your head is being lifted away from your body, and your neck is stretching. It feels relaxed and good.

3 Focus on your shoulder muscles. These huge muscles play a tremendous role in keeping your head upright, and they can get very tense. Let them relax. You should feel some tingling or burning sensations in the upper back and shoulder muscles. You can feel the muscles ease.

4 Imagine your muscles are contracted to perform a certain exercise and you are now trying to extend and relax these muscles to do the exact opposite. Similarly let the shoulders relax. The region is expanding now and the tension is going away. Your biceps are elongating, they are stretching and relaxing. All the muscles in your upper arms that are used to pull and push are relaxing.

5 Now focus on your hands. Feel the release of tension, particularly in the hand you use most. Feel the fingers relax and a tingling sensation as the blood rushes to the tips of your fingers. All the smaller muscles between the bones in your hand are relaxing. Your hands feel energised.

6 Concentrate on your upper back. See in your mind the muscles stretching, all the tension dissipating. Tension has caused your spine to shrink and tighten. Feel it elongating as your muscles relax. Your buttock muscles on which you have been sitting have become very tight. Expand them, let the blood go into them. Feel them relax.

7 Focus on your hamstrings. Feel them relax. The muscles in your legs and the back of your thighs are loosening. Feel warm as they relax and rest. Your shin and calf muscles have become congested from sitting upright. Imagine all the tension going and the blood flowing upwards, passively. Feel your heels relaxing, the soles of your feet relaxing. You have taken your shoes off, you see the blood rushing towards your toes. Feel that tingling sensation in your toes. Your body feels very relaxed.

8 Focus on your jaws and temples. Tension creates a biting reflex. Now let the jaws relax. The temples relax. Feel your eyebrows relax. Your eyelids feel very heavy. You have to keep your eyes wide open. They were tense from looking at your work, from focusing on particular spots. Now you are letting your inner eye muscles relax. Let the eye muscles and the balls of your eyes relax. Your throat and your lips are relaxing. Let your mouth and throat muscles and the muscles in the rest of your face relax.

You are now completely relaxed.

the early years

Our tastes change and mature as we grow up, but basic eating habits established in childhood can stay with us for life. What young children eat is mostly decided by adults – parents or guardians, friends' parents, school staff etc. – so it is our duty to introduce them to the right sort of foods and to teach them about nutrition. To a great extent we have lost the traditional wisdom passed on from parents to children; it was an excellent tradition and should never have been sidelined.

Babies and very young children need a diet that is carefully formulated to suit their needs. Once children sit up at the table and eat with the rest of the family, and particularly once they have reached the age of about ten, try to make a rule of catering for all the family together.

babies

Before he or she is born, a baby's supply of nutrients has come via the placenta, the lining of its mother's womb. Although it may have swallowed some amniotic fluid while swimming in it in the mother's womb, it has had no need to breathe, eat or drink. As soon as it is born, however, its early life will be filled with little else.

There is no doubt that the best food for a new baby is mother's milk. This milk is exactly like plasma (blood minus the red blood cells), and is very high in protein. In some places special cheese is made out of the milk of the cow in the first few days after delivery of the calf. (Some say it is delicious but I think that it is depriving the calf, who needs every drop of it.)

A mother's milk has everything that a very young baby needs: protein, glucose to help with its high energy demand, minerals, vitamins, fluids and immune particles to defend against infections. The demand for fluids and nutrients is so high that a baby will need to feed every couple of hours throughout the day and part of the night.

If a mother is unable to breastfeed, her baby will have to be given processed or 'formula' milk. Claims are made about this being the next best thing after mother's milk, but it is as far away from nature as it could be. I have found it can cause inflamed and itchy patches around the mouth, cheeks and the anal region, the very areas the milk is in contact with, which may well be an indication that not all is well.

Breast milk will be affected by what the mother herself eats, so while breastfeeding I suggest you avoid excess garlic, spicy foods, mangoes, pineapples, salt, yeast products and chocolate, and steer clear of canned or preserved foods (for the chemicals or preservatives), alcohol, coffee and bottled drinks containing caffeine or artificial sweeteners. You may need vitamin and mineral supplements, but do not take these unnecessarily. Also avoid antibiotics, contraceptive pills, steroids, weight-control pills, antidepressants, recreational drugs and smoking.

A baby grows at a phenomenal rate, roughly 200 g a day for the first few weeks. A baby should receive exclusively, day and night, breast milk and water for about three to four months. Then cow's milk and semi-solid food can be introduced two to four times a day. This will reduce the demand for mother's milk.

first foods

Babies have a very sensitive gut lining and new foods should be introduced slowly. Until about six months a baby's diet will continue to be largely milk but with the gradual addition of purées and juices. (For a baby being fed on formula milk it is advisable to begin this a little earlier, rather than continue with processed or artificial milk; the baby's development will benefit from the additional nourishment.) If your baby demands food all the time by crying, move on to the next phase of feeding.

From about four months, start supplementing milk feeds with some baked apple, thoroughly mashed up, and baby rice. The process of baking retains most of the nutrients but the heat destroys the enzymes in fruit and fruit juices that are too powerful for a baby's gut lining. Once the baby gets used to baked apple, introduce puréed vegetables (again, cooked to neutralise the raw enzymes). Semi-solid purées like this are more easily swallowed than liquids, which may cause

choking. Next, move on to soups. Boil vegetables like cabbage, carrots, peas and potatoes in a salt-free chicken stock. Blend the soup until smooth and give it when tepid in a baby cup with a nozzle.

Around five months you can start to introduce juices. Start with fresh carrot or apple juice, just a few spoonfuls in the beginning, to allow the baby's system to adjust. Other introductory foods that go down well at this stage are:
• Mashed bananas.
• Plums and seedless grapes, squashed to a pulp.
• Oat and digestive biscuits soaked in water, fed with a spoon (this will help with learning to swallow).

These early foods will prepare the baby for the first solid food, at about six months (five months if the baby is not breastfed or was born prematurely and fed on formula milk). In Bengal there is a celebration when the baby reaches six months and is given its first solid food, in the form of rice pudding – the entire family gathers for a feast, bringing new clothes and gifts, and watches the baby eat for the first time.

An easy to digest but really nourishing first food is kichri rice. Give this once a day for a few days and then twice a day. Rice pudding is also a good option, with a little mashed banana to sweeten it.

kichri rice

Soak half a cup of lentils (yellow dahl) for 2–4 hours, changing the water a couple of times. Rinse thoroughly to make sure that no powdery residue remains.

Thoroughly wash half a cup of good-quality long-grain rice.

Put the lentils and rice into a saucepan. Add 4 cups of water and a pinch of turmeric (optional) and 1 teaspoon of olive oil. Boil the mixture until it thickens and then cook slowly until it becomes mushy. Add more

water, if necessary, to ensure the lentils are soft, then boil to drive off any excess water. Stir thoroughly and leave until it is just warm.

Salt-free chicken or lamb stock, instead of water, will make this mixture rich in peptones (refined protein) and minerals (calcium, magnesium etc. for the bones), making it especially nourishing for prematurely born babies and those who haven't been breastfed for more than a month.

bananas

Much loved by young children, bananas are highly nutritious. They provide fibre and carbohydrate, vitamins (especially B_6), potassium, calcium, iron, zinc and folic acid. Ripe bananas contain enzymes that aid digestion; they are good for treating diarrhoea as they act as a stool binder as well as an antimicrobial agent. In addition, they have antibacterial properties – the insides of banana skins are often rubbed on cuts and wounds to disinfect them. With all these qualities, it is no wonder that bananas are offered to the gods in Hindu religious ceremonies.

Soft-boiled eggs are a good source of proteins at this age and are usually a favourite with babies. Choose free-range eggs from a reliable source. Boil the egg for two minutes, scoop out the egg from the shell with a spoon and mash, making sure there are no fragments of shell.

Continue breastfeeding a few times a day as you introduce these other foods. In an ideal situation you can continue breastfeeding periodically until nine months or even a year. By this time it becomes comfort food rather than a necessity, and later it can become increasingly difficult to wean a baby off mother's milk, as suckling becomes a habit.

A baby's first teeth start to appear at around four months. (A baby's age in months minus 2 gives you an indication as to how many teeth a baby should have at any stage, so at eight months you can expect six teeth.) Once six teeth have appeared, a baby can manage minced chicken or turkey. Although these first teeth are not used to bite or grind in the early stages, training them is a good idea. Boil the mince for 30 minutes, then mix it with puréed vegetables, mashed potatoes, overcooked rice or kichri rice. Serve it first for lunch and then in the evenings. Once you have established solid food for the final meal of the day, the baby will not need milk at night but may still cry because of thirst, to which water is the answer.

The demand for energy increases hugely as babies learn to kick, giggle and wave. Exercising all the time they are awake develops muscle tone, enabling them to first hold their heads up, then sit, crawl, stand and finally walk. By the end of the first year a baby will have trebled in weight to around 10 kg.

what to avoid

There are a few foods that are not suitable for babies. These include:
• Salt. It's easy to forget that stocks and gravy are often high in salt. If you add salt to vegetables for the rest of the family, keep your baby's share separate.
• Orange juice. This is too acid for a young stomach, and also contributes to nappy rash and rashes on the cheeks. Apple and grape juices are much better 'starter juices'. You can then introduce the occasional orange juice, but in the form of freshly squeezed juice from a sweet variety of clementine or tangerine diluted with water or mixed with a little carrot juice (which is naturally alkaline).

toddlers

Once a child has begun to walk, the demand for food naturally increases. Walking speeds the development of bones, so weight gain is rapid. Food by this time should consist of soups, juices and easily digestible solid meals such as fish cakes, minced meat or chicken, mashed vegetables or potatoes, rice and porridge, with biscuits to gnaw on. This is a good time to invest in kitchen appliances such as a juicer, chopper and blender, as they will soon be in frequent use.

Once a child has enough teeth to chew food well – the set of baby teeth is nearly complete by 15–18 months – meals should be more varied and include more solid food (see illustration). Lunch and dinner can include pasta, vegetables (well cooked or steamed) and boneless fish and meat. Unless your child has an intolerance to cow's or goat's milk, offer milk twice a day: a glass after breakfast and another at bedtime (about 2 hours after supper). Chilled milk slows down the digestive process, often causing gases and abdominal colic, so warm the milk and, if it makes it more palatable, sweeten it with a little honey. A strand or two of saffron infused in the milk acts as a good tonic for a child who looks pale and whose hair is very thin.

In the first year of a baby's life paediatricians are particularly concerned about weight and they always weigh the baby at the beginning of a visit. After that, once a baby begins to walk, weight is suddenly less of an issue, unless a toddler is seriously under- or overweight.

At the age of two a child should weigh around 20 kg. Children develop very quickly at this stage, so a heavier child may not necessarily be of concern, but do apply a common-sense approach even at

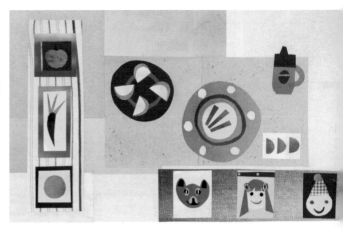

this early age and seek a professional nutritionist's advice if you feel your toddler is overweight.

Introducing eating habits at mealtimes, even at this early stage, may help avoid later problems:
• Feed a toddler slowly, and slow them down periodically with sips of water. This will be more time-consuming for you, but someone in the habit of eating rapidly is also inclined to eat too much.
• Massage the neck and shoulders at bedtime. This improves blood flow to the brain and will help the appetite centre to control the demand for food, helpful both to gorgers and those who eat too little.
• Once or twice a week, to allow the stomach a little rest, give just rice pudding for supper. Even if

ideas for toddler meals

• Lamb or beef and vegetable casserole, plus mashed potatoes or rice.
• Minced chicken cooked with a little garlic, olive oil, fresh tomatoes and peas, served with rice or egg noodles. Boil noodles separately then mix the two together.
• Home-made spaghetti bolognese made with fresh chopped tomatoes, mixed herbs and minced meat.
• Shepherd's or cottage pie. This is a good way of introducing carrots, leeks, peas and onion, which can all be added to the minced meat.

• Kebabs (see page 76) with rice or mashed potatoes and steamed vegetables.
• Some tender, well-done meat from the Sunday roast with vegetables and potatoes, a good way of bringing a toddler into family meals.
• Home-made fish cakes, made with boneless mashed fish rolled in breadcrumbs.
• Mango or other fruit purées, fruit salad and baked apple all make tasty and nourishing puddings, but leave them until about an hour after the main course is finished.

toddler kebabs

250 g minced meat
a little garlic
a little ginger paste
1 egg

Mix the meat, garlic and ginger together thoroughly. Lightly beat the egg and add half to the meat mixture. Mix well then leave for 10–15 minutes for the flavours to mingle. Roll the meat into 5–6 sausage shapes and put a skewer through each. Grill, turning them as they brown, until cooked through.

your child is skinny or underweight, a light meal every now and then doesn't affect the weight, as the body will make up for it at other times.
• Try to cater for the family all together. There may be specific dietary requirements that make this difficult, but except in those cases, struggling to provide several tailor-made meals both encourages fads and makes life a lot more difficult – and it's when you feel that there is not enough time that you are more likely to fall back on convenience foods.

Six meals a day
Toddlers up to the age of two should eat about six times a day, as follows:
Breakfast: porridge or cereal, soft boiled egg, fresh fruit juice.
Mid-morning: warm milk and biscuits.
Lunch: a mixture of protein, carbohydrates and vegetables.
Mid-afternoon (4 pm): fruit or vegetable juice, fruit or a fruity milkshake.
Supper (6 pm): as lunch, but a slightly smaller portion.
Bedtime (8 pm): milk with honey or malt drink in milk.

learning to enjoy vegetables ...
A diet of meat and starch with no greens or fresh fruit is as unhealthy a diet as one can have. Fruit and vegetables are vital sources of vitamins and minerals, as well as providing fibre to facilitate bowel movements, keeping young digestive systems in good order. But vegetables, in particular, are often a source of pet hates. Once children start school they will be highly influenced by their school friends' fads and fancies, so introduce a wide range of vegetables early on, to develop a taste for them before peer pressure takes over. Don't let your own dislikes show, either, as children very quickly pick up on these and imitate them. We all have food prejudices, often set in our own childhood, but they should not be perpetuated from generation to generation.

Some of the popular 'hate' vegetables have gained their reputation by being badly cooked and poorly presented. First impressions count for a lot.

Brassicas Cabbages, cauliflowers and their relations give off a smell when cooking that not even the most ardent cabbage-lover would describe as pleasant (Brussels sprouts are the worst) and this has turned many people of all ages off eating them. Drop a bay leaf or two and a cinnamon stick into the cooking water to neutralise the cabbagy smell and help avoid the connection between smell and taste.

The fibrous, woody stems of broccoli can be offputting. Divide the heads into small, individual florets and the 'little trees' will have much more appeal. Cauliflower is also more attractive in small florets, but the pallid colour doesn't look appetising. If this is a problem, use cauliflower in vegetable soups, where it purées well and contributes goodness without announcing its presence.

Spinach If your early experience of spinach is as a slimy mass with a trickle of thin green water oozing from it, you are not likely to take to it. The central ribs take longer to cook, by which time the soft leaves will be overcooked, so strip the stalks away and just allow the leaves to wilt for a minute or two. Squeeze out well. Spinach goes particularly well with egg: try chopping some raw leaves very finely and stirring them into scrambled or mashed hardboiled eggs.

Beetroot This is a rich source of minerals, especially potassium, and it is very good for mild constipation in children. Choose small beets, the size of golf balls, and bake them until cooked through (the skin will then come off easily). Or try a little grated raw beetroot mixed with grated carrot for a really vibrant combination.

Root vegetables Lifelong dislikes of parsnips and turnips have been triggered by old, woody specimens that have either got hard centres (which survive as lumps even when mashed) or that have been overcooked to a mush that is neither tasty nor nutritious. So make your children's introduction to them a much more palatable one – small, young roots will be tender and have a natural sweetness that most children crave. They purée easily and add interest to the blandness of mashed potato; swede and carrots also add colour.

Of course, taste is a very personal thing and there are sure to be certain foods that your child truly does not like. Don't force the issue – meals should not become a time of misery or test of wills – but try a rejected vegetable on several different occasions, prepared in various ways before crossing it off the list. We have a greater choice of foods than ever before, so there is no need to get stuck in an unimaginative 'peas, beans or carrots' rut.

That said, these everyday vegetables are good sources of essential nutrients. Carrots, which are a good source of carotene, a form of vitamin A needed by the eyes, are particularly versatile. As well as being served plain, they mash well with potatoes or other root vegetables and can also be juiced. Carrot juice blended with apple juice makes a very palatable drink.

... and fruit

Citrus fruit have a 'healthy' reputation, but the citric acid they contain means not all of them are good news (see page 41). As far as possible, avoid giving toddlers orange and grapefruit juices, although note the fibres in the whole unjuiced fruit are alkaline and neutralise some of the acid. Choose sweet varieties such as tangerine, satsuma or pink grapefruit (taste it yourself first) and limit them to two fruits a week.

As well as apples, pears and bananas (often a favourite), ring the changes with other fruit as it comes into season – cherries (stoned and chopped), apricots, peaches and nectarines, melon – and exotics like kiwi and papaya (ideal for constipation).

food intolerances and allergies

Most parents are alert to violent reactions to certain well-known allergens, such as nuts, but may not always associate lesser symptoms like bloating, insomnia or periodic nappy rash to a food sensitivity. If you suspect a pattern of cause and effect, eliminate the suspected food items and see if the complaint disappears. See also pages 197–8.

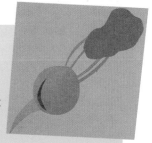

beetroot

Rich in vitamin A, folic acid, potassium and manganese, beetroot is a very good remedy for constipation. Beetroot is also credited in some societies with cancer-fighting properties. Sadly, too many people know beetroot only as tart, vinegary slices or cubes in bottles. From a child's point of view, however, here is something with an interesting colour and, when young, a very sweet taste.

after-school snacks

Children are often ravenous when they get home from school. Sidetrack them from the sweet shop or the cake tin with some of these:

• Vegetable fingers with a variety of dips. Try cottage cheese, hummus, tzatziki or sour cream with chives. Baby carrots, celery sticks and cucumber strips also get them eating fresh raw vegetables.

• Potato cakes. Mash potatoes with a little butter or olive oil and a pinch of salt. Shape into flattened cakes about 1 cm thick (the children can help with this), then roll in a thin coating of flour to help prevent the cakes from breaking up while cooking. Fry them gently in olive oil until a thin golden crust is formed.

• Corn on the cob.

• A bowl of fresh fruit salad (apples, grapes, melon, kiwi) dressed with honey, thick creamy yoghurt or even a little low-fat fresh cream.

• Kebab cakes. Soak 250 g of chickpeas overnight. Boil with 500 g of minced meat, garlic, chopped ginger and a little salt to taste until the chickpeas are soft and the water has boiled away (this takes an hour or so). Leave to cool, then stir in a raw egg to make a firm paste. Make golf-ball-sized balls of the mixture and flatten them into discs. Fry in olive oil on a medium heat until they turn light brown. They make a filling, healthy snack and freeze well; defrost before frying.

fast track

Fast foods, from ready-prepared just-heat-and-serve-meals to takeaway burgers, appeal not only to children but to busy parents run off their feet and looking for an easy option. The danger of these is threefold:

• You do not know exactly what you are feeding your children – the ingredients list may detail a certain percentage of fish or meat, but it tells you nothing about the quality. What constitutes fish and meat in labelling terms is wider than you would expect and almost certainly wider than you would find acceptable from the local butcher or fishmonger.

• Pre-prepared food is generally much higher in salt and sugar than home-cooked food (see page 44), training young palates to yearn for sugar and salt.

• To give food a respectable shelf life, preservatives need to be added. Although government food regulations require that these are not present in harmful quantities, this does not take account of accumulations in the system or unforeseen long-term complications. Announcements are regularly made either banning or further limiting food additives, which brings into question what these additives might already have done.

So, avoid all fast foods, however convenient they may be. The long-term health of your children rests on early nutrition and you should take time to ensure that your children eat healthily right from the beginning. Miss this opportunity, and your children will grow up eating only convenience food, to their permanent detriment. There are some good-quality prepared products available, but to save time you will first need to spend some time learning to interpret what labels actually mean (see pages 47–8) and what different methods of preserving do to food (see page 49).

The good news is that not all fast, convenient food is a fast food or a convenience food:

• It takes no more time to grill a fresh fillet of fish as it does to defrost and cook fish fingers.

• Putting a potato in the oven to bake is less work than reheating a ready meal – and it doesn't even need unwrapping. (Put a metal skewer through the centre of the potato and it will cut the cooking time, too.)

• When making a stew or casserole, make two or three times as much and freeze the extra as individual portions, ready to be defrosted and eaten with minimal further work.

• Long, slow-cooked dishes can be prepared many hours ahead. Get them ready at a time convenient to you and leave them to their own devices – with such gentle cooking an hour or two more or less will not make any difference, and will take the pressure off a busy timetable.

As they get a little older, engage children's interest in cooking. There is no entertainment value in taking a plastic sleeve off a ready-cooked meal and watching it revolve in the microwave, but they will enjoy weighing out ingredients and mixing them together, pressing the button on a chopping or blending machine and making 'shaped' food like fish cakes and kebabs.

Home-made versions of fast food make good occasional treats. Make your own pizzas and you can control what goes on them – children have great fun choosing and arranging their own toppings. A beefburger made with good-quality meat minced at home will spoil the taste of flat, pappy apologies of commercial burgers for the whole family. (Also see page 83.)

sweets and treats

All children are tempted by sweets, ice creams and fizzy drinks. Some chemicals in these can be addictive or mood-changing for some children, so be very careful how you handle them. Rather than

hyperactivity and diet

Food can affect mood and behaviour, and susceptible children can react dramatically.

Hyperactivity is akin to an allergy, but one where the result is a mental rather than a physical eruption (see pages 197–8 for more information on the manifestation of allergies). Hyperactive children are disruptive in class and unsettling to family life; they also upset and scare themselves by their inability to stop. Not every fidgety child who won't concentrate is suffering from ADHD (attention deficit hyperactivity disorder), but spotting correlations between certain foods and behaviour patterns can be helpful for all children.

There are degrees of sensitivity and triggers differ from person to person. Common ones include sugar, caffeine and food additives, especially colourings such as tartrazine (yellow). Some children respond badly to everyday foods such as strawberries.

Excess sugar or caffeine gives an injection of short-term energy followed by a low, so moderate children's intake of:
• Sweets.
• Fizzy drinks, especially colas.
• Cakes and sugary biscuits.
• Ice cream.
• Condensed milk.
• Gums.
• Chocolate.

Susceptible children will be able to cope with less before they become 'manic', and some can be set off by even small amounts, such as the syrup used for children's cough mixtures and medicines.

A hyperactive child often sleeps poorly. To induce more restful sleep, try the following:
• Give a neck and spine massage at bedtime two or three times a week.
• Make sure they do not play exciting video games or watch disturbing TV programmes in the evening (nature films often appeal most as a substitute).
• Evening walks will use up energy without over-exciting the way a game of football or chasing around might.
• Teach them a few relaxing yoga postures. It can also be useful to train children to observe a period of silence (from 15 minutes to 1 hour a day).
• Nurture an interest in absorbing but peaceful activities such as drawing and music.

for healthy young teeth and gums

In addition to regular brushing of teeth in the morning and at bedtime, biting and chewing crunchy fruit and vegetables such as apples and raw carrots will help to strengthen young teeth and gums.

A good supply of calcium is vital to the healthy development of teeth and bones: see pages 18 and 20 for information on milk and additional sources of calcium.

Teach children to rinse and gargle after each meal so that particles of food, particularly meat fibres, are washed out.

Don't allow them to eat anything sweet after brushing at night.

ban them entirely, which can raise them to the status of forbidden fruits, let them remain as occasional treats. Don't make them rewards to be worked for, and make it clear that they are special treats and do not in any way replace meals.

When most meals are healthy and nutritious, a few can afford to break the rules. Serve the 'naughty' things only rarely and in moderation – buy or make just enough rich chocolate cake or ice cream, for instance, to be consumed at one time – and children can relish them without their bodies becoming upset. If nearly every meal included things like chips and ice cream, then the body's ability to digest and neutralise the ill-effects would be undermined. Furthermore, it would build the habit of bad eating which would last not only through childhood, but their entire lives.

puppy fat

Fat children can be given a hard time by their peers, especially if their size makes them the odd one out (children can be very unforgiving about anything outside their perceived norm) or hampers their ability at sports and games. Do not nag or criticise them, which may make them turn to food for comfort. In addition to ensuring they do not eat too much, or too many of the wrong things, there are several things that can help:
• Teach children to eat slowly (the appetite centre then has time to send the 'enough' message to the brain before they eat too much).
• Acid is an appetite stimulant, so avoid citrus fruits, fizzy drinks (which contain citric acid as a preservative), vinegar, nuts and spicy food.
• Say no to snacks between meals.
• Refrain from providing sweets or food (except a piece of fruit) for an hour before bedtime.
• Eat with them. Eating alone, they will be more inclined to eat faster and raid the kitchen for more food. Seize opportune moments at mealtimes to explain healthy eating.

There is general concern over how inactive many children are, and exercise is a vital part of avoiding becoming overweight, or of losing weight. Take a look at how much exercise your child gets – this does not have to be formal sports or exercise classes, but walking, swimming and generally playing active games. For overweight children, especially, these are probably more acceptable than organised sport, so incorporate regular walks into family life; play impromptu ball games together or get in the habit of going swimming at the weekend.

Some children, far from being couch potatoes, are hyperactive – forever restless, unable to stay concentrated on one task for more than a few minutes, agitated to the point of exhaustion. Elements in the diet can be a contributory factor to this (see page 81).

when children fall sick

Schools are notorious as places where colds and coughs spread like wildfire. When I see a child who is prey to one minor ailment after another, showing signs of a weak immune system, I very often recommend Regimen Therapy alone (see chapter 7), without even a drop of vitamins or minerals. Children respond so well that all they often need is simple assistance like this. Most children's coughs and colds are viral in origin, so antibiotics have no role to play.

You can help to guard your children against colds and flu, especially during winter and early spring when these viruses are particularly prevalent (see pages 162–6), by following these guidelines:
• Offer chicken soup and lamb broth, which provide lots of useful minerals and proteins.
• Give them carrot and apple juice, which are good sources of vitamins.
• Avoid ice cream and chilled drinks (particularly fizzy drinks) as they harm the throat.
• Too much cheese produces more mucus in the sinuses, and when these get filled up the dripping nose starts. The excess mucus is a breeding ground for infections in the throat and sinuses.

If a cold or flu virus gets past these defences, let your children rest in bed for one or two days, drinking soup and water. Comfort and build up their reserves with:

• Fresh chicken soup – nutritious but not energy-sapping.
• Liquorice tea with honey: 1–2 cups daily for a week.
• 1–2 drops of sinus oil in each nostril twice daily.
• A gentle throat massage with a mentholated cream or vapour rub.
• A neck and shoulder massage with Dr Ali's Junior Massage oil, a mixture of sweet almond, eucalyptus and lavender (see page 220).

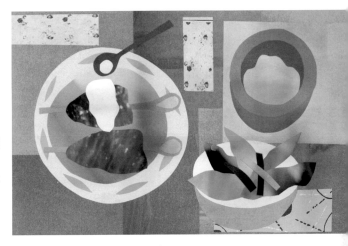

home-style fast food

To entice your teenager away from junk food, reproduce the best fast-food favourites with healthier alternatives:
• Jacket potatoes with a chilli mince topping.
• Corn on the cob with a little melted butter, salt and pepper to taste and a few drops of lemon juice.
• Tortilla wraps with a range of fillings: cooked chicken or turkey, sliced sweet peppers, salad, hummus or Mexican mashed beans.
• Grilled kebabs made with good-quality mince, with a spicy tomato sauce or a Greek-style yoghurt and cucumber dip and a big bowl of salad (see illustration above).

Introduce some fast food of your own:
• Fish cakes well flavoured with garlic, pepper and coriander or parsley.

• Pancakes with different fillings: smoked salmon and dill; garlicky minced meat; or go Chinese with shredded duck and stir-fried mixed vegetables.
• Fried golf balls. Make fillings of mashed potato mixed with either mixed vegetables and nuts, minced meat, or boiled and mashed egg, seasoned well. Shape into 'golf balls'. Cut the crusts off bread (two slices per ball), dampen and seal the balls in a bread overcoat. Fry, drain well and eat hot.

To make a break from colas and fizzy drinks, ring the changes with:
• Home-made squashes.
• Iced tea.
• Exotic juices.
• Milk shakes.
• Ice cream shakes (vanilla ice cream mixed with fruit syrup and soda water).

store cupboard staples for teenage snackers

An attack of the munchies can be assuaged either by a shot of sugar (a handful of dried fruit rather than a spoonful of sugar) which will signal to the brain to release glycogen stored in the liver, or by dampening the stimulation of stomach acid with plain oat biscuits, a glass of cold milk or even a glass of water. Instant access is important, so make alternatives to cakes and cans readily available. Here are some suggestions for healthy snacks.

instead of …
- Rich, creamy cakes.
- Sweets and chocolates.
- Crisps.
- Fizzy drinks, especially 'energy' drinks.

try …
- Biscuits low in sugar and butter (check the labels).
- 'Pop-in-the-mouth' fruit like grapes, cherries, physalis.
- Nuts, ready shelled and preferably unsalted.
- Fruit juices, hi-juice drinks and flavoured mineral water.

the teens

Teenagers, it seems, have traditionally always eaten badly. Nearly 2000 years ago Galen, the great Greek surgeon-physician, was describing youths as having a tendency to eat anything they could lay their hands on and were able to digest it without any serious health complications.

Ensuring teenagers eat healthily can be problematic, but parents can also worry themselves unnecessarily. A good diet for the first twelve or fifteen years of their lives will have built up a healthy constitution and puberty brings on a burst of hormones that, like a pregnant woman, enables teenagers to eat and digest food that might cause problems for older and younger generations. Testing boundaries and learning to make decisions for themselves is all part of becoming independent, and allowing food to become a battleground is more likely to cause problems than resolve them. What is important is that you keep in touch with your children through this period. Talk to them about all sorts of things, what they enjoy and what they worry about (without them feeling you are prying or mollycoddling), get to know their friends, and how they pass their time. Pressures, emotional confusion and unhappiness are often reflected in appetite and eating habits, and being alert to these at an early stage is important in averting major problems such as eating disorders or seriously poor nutrition.

countering the effects of junk food

When out with friends, the lure of greasy, oversweet and caffeine-laden foods and drinks will probably be irresistible to teenagers. Forgoing the burgers and fries that everyone else has in favour of a salad would be tantamount to admitting to going to bed early or choosing a style of shoe because it is sensible.

At home, therefore, make every effort to offer them healthy food, particularly fruit and salad. This will be easier if you have set a good eating regime when they were younger. Avoid stocking foods that are prepacked or canned; citrus juices (they stimulate appetite); fizzy drinks and snacks high in yeast, fats or sugars. Introduce them to herbal teas and encourage them to drink at least six big glasses of water a day.

Start the day with a breakfast of cereals, milk, eggs and soda bread toast and see that they get a good hot meal once a day whenever possible. It will help if you set a regular pattern to meals, rather than members of the family all catering for themselves and 'grazing' when they want. Encourage them to eat slowly and try to see they don't eat too many acid-producing foods (fried food, colas, nuts, spicy food and tomato ketchup as well as citrus fruit), as excess stomach acid creates a voracious appetite.

Much of the appeal of fast food (apart from the social aspect) is the strong flavourings and variety rather than the actual speed of delivery – the taste of fried food and highly spiced coatings and sauces have overwhelmed and retrained teenage taste buds. Think how this could be reinterpreted into a healthier alternative at home; limit the money they have with which to eat out, and home food will regain its attractions.

Imposing rules with an iron will is likely to be met with mutiny and rebellion, but it is good child psychology, and indeed the truth, to tell them that junk food will affect their skin, bring out more acne, give them headaches or allergies, and that they need the calcium and fresh foods for their growing pains. Also, keep attuned to who they admire and adulate – being able to point out that a particular film or pop star advocates a healthy diet is a useful armament to have.

coping with growing up

When children reach puberty their dietary requirements change. Good supplies of protein, minerals and vitamins are very important: they are growing in height, are very active and their reproductive hormones are carrying out very sophisticated work.

Teenagers, particularly boys, can develop formidable appetites. This is not really surprising. They are growing fast, developing muscle and changing shape. They are expending a huge amount of mental effort, both in their studies and in coping with emotional and hormonal turmoil. They are using up a lot of physical energy with sports, and on top of this perhaps staying up late, dancing to all hours, and yet are still full of nervous energy. All this needs a lot of fuel. So they will eat prodigious amounts and sleep long hours to compensate.

All this change and growth can also have the opposite effect. Living up to a supposed ideal body shape can lead to teenagers, especially but not exclusively girls, being hypercritical about their own bodies. Peer pressure and the glamorous images of the media encourage this dissatisfaction, which can begin as early as 11 or 12, and can result in eating too little and flirting with unsuitable diets.

There are psychological pressures at work too. Getting very thin can in some be not a fashion statement but a way of staving off impending adulthood, with its pressures and responsibilities. Amenorrhea (cessation of menstrual periods), anorexia and bulimia are all extreme but unfortunately not rare conditions (see pages 87–9 and 217).

Many girls and boys suddenly put on weight at puberty. An endocrinological check-up may reveal

apricots

When I spent a few days with a little-known tribe high in the Himalayas, I was amazed to see how precious apricots were to them. They believed they gave them longevity (many of the villagers were over 100 years old). The kernel provided fuel and cooking oil, while the flesh of the fruit provided vitamins and minerals (especially zinc and iron) and useful protein. Dried apricots do not attract bacteria because the skin has antibacterial properties, and during the long winter months, dried apricots are a great source of vitamins and minerals. The high fibre content eases bowel movements, and apricot oil has anti-inflammatory properties, both when rubbed into joints or taken internally.

whether hormones are causing the weight increase. Diet is part of the solution, but an experienced cranial osteopath and massage of the neck and shoulder area can improve cranial circulation and improve functions of the hypothalamus, which controls appetite, and the pituitary, which controls hormones of the thyroid gland, the main metabolic controller. Deep-seated problems such as parental conflict, bullying in school or loneliness can cause binge eating. Don't criticise or mock an overweight teenager – self-esteem is fragile at this age – but it is important to find out whether the cause is hormonal, a compensation for unhappiness or simple over-eating.

Once menstruation begins, girls will need to make sure they are getting sufficient iron. Although there is no actual loss of circulating blood during a period, many teenage girls are slightly anaemic. Good sources of iron include:
• Red meat and offal.
• Eggs.
• 'Fortified' breakfast cereals.
• Pulses and lentils.
• Dried apricots.
• Dark green leafy vegetables.

Iron from a non-animal source needs the help of vitamin C to be absorbed (usefully it is also often present in the same food as long as it hasn't leached out through cooking – see pages 52–5), while tea, coffee and colas inhibit absorption, so sometimes it is more than just the actual source of iron that needs boosting.

A rampant sex drive with no satisfactory source of release is immensely frustrating for younger teenagers. Eggs, excess red meat, garlic, ginger, saffron, excess sugar (from chocolates and fizzy drinks) caffeine and excess salt are all 'hot' foods that fire up the hormones and may send young boys into overdrive. In ancient times, tukmaria seeds or the fresh leaves of cumin, anise, mint or poppy, all 'cooling' herbs and spices, were used in cooking or as an infusion and fed to sexually hyperactive young lads! This balance of cooling and heating foods can still be followed today (see pages 38–9).

Acne is a major problem for many teenagers. The standard treatment is to prescribe strong antibiotics for months (often damaging the liver and kidneys) until bacteria finally give up. The sensible way to treat it is through proper eating – see pages 180–81.

the teenage vegetarian

This is not about growing up in a vegetarian family, but about teenagers who decide peremptorily to give up meat.

A strict vegetarian diet in puberty or during a growing phase is not a good idea, but do not nag or use harsh words of criticism. This will be counter-productive. Be compassionate and use logic. Support their stance and the good intentions behind it, but explain that it becomes even more important that they take care of what they eat. Vegetarians are in danger of missing out on two types of vital nutrition:
• Some of the amino acids essential for building protein (muscles) in the body. Lack of protein in the system can cause low blood pressure and even anaemia. This will lead to tiredness and more colds and coughs due to a weakened immune system.
• Fat-soluble vitamins like A, D, E and K. We get these from animal fats (calling them 'lipids' may take away unwelcome 'fat' connotations). During puberty vitamins E and D are very important in helping with hormonal balance, skin and bone development (calcium absorption is facilitated by vitamin D). Acne is liable to worsen if the body is short of these vitamins, and lack of vitamin E can trigger period problems in girls.

Also, a move to a pure vegetable diet denies you the full satisfaction of eating what you are used to, so new vegetarians are inclined to try to make up for this by eating lots of cheese, sweets and snacks, which are unhealthy in excess.

Let them think through for themselves what all this means. Much will depend on their reasons for embracing vegetarianism. Animal rights campaigns, a new awareness of how food is produced or peer pressure (again) turn many a

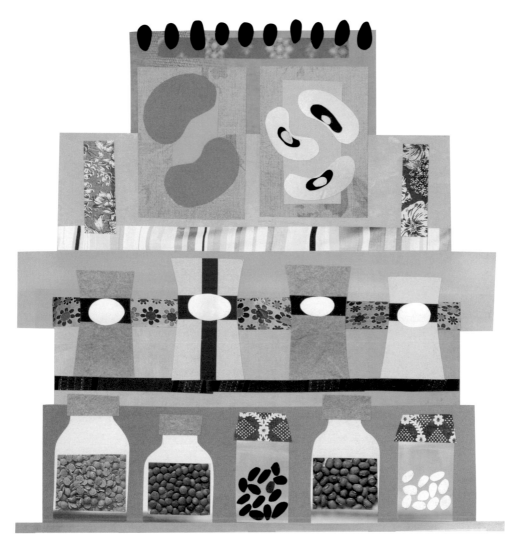

teenager off meat and they may campaign aggressively for everybody in the family to do the same. Alternatively the reason (perhaps masked by an interest in animal welfare) may be an effort to lose weight or a symptom of deeper problems.

If altruistic motivation leads a young person to think about nutrition and to question methods of food production, then it will be a useful (probably temporary) experience and all you need do is ensure they are getting all the nutrition they need. See pages 36–8 for advice on a balanced vegetarian diet and illustration (above). If, however, the change seems self-centred and results in eating very little, be alert to more worrying underlying causes such as anorexia.

anorexia and bulimia

These eating disorders are not the exclusive domain of teenagers, but teenage girls certainly form by far the largest group (for more information see page 217). Some of the recognisable signs of anorexia include:

• Suddenly becoming vegetarian or vegan.
• Eating much less – avoiding butter, cheese and most carbohydrates but craving salads.
• Jogging or exercising a lot.
• Becoming very elusive and egocentric.
• Hating to be criticised for anything.

However, these are also behaviour traits of a lot of teenagers not in the slightest danger of becoming anorexic. Be alert to signs of trouble by knowing your teenager, and consider also:

• Do they deny they are not eating enough? If they avoid meals by saying they have already eaten at a friend's, check this out.

• Are they getting secret support via the Internet? A great deal of inaccurate information is presented as fact on websites – there is no vetting or control of these – and via chat rooms fellow anorexics may be undoing all the progress being made on other fronts.

• Are they obsessed with their weight and shape, even though they are not fat?

• Do they vomit on a regular basis or spend a lot of time in the toilet after meals?

• Is there evidence of them taking laxatives or diuretics?

Although these are psychological disorders, there is a lot one can do nutritionally.

anorexia

Given a choice, anorexics would live on, at most, lettuce and steamed vegetables. To an anorexic, the main 'enemies' are flesh, fats and sweet, sugary things. While you can pass on the sweet foods, the missed proteins and fat-soluble vitamins are essential, so concentrate on these. Do not force them to eat such overtly meaty/fatty foods as chicken, fish or cheese, but provide high-nutrition, low-fuss foods such as:

• Soaked almonds.

• Ghee in rice, lentils or soup.

• Bean sprouts (sprout them yourself at home so they can be eaten when newly sprouted, when the protein levels are at their highest).

• Avocado.

• Jacket potatoes (olive oil rather than butter or cheese may make these appear more acceptable).

• Lentils and beans.

• Rice.

• Soya or tofu preparations.

• Cottage cheese.

• Pomegranate.

• Carrot and apple juice.

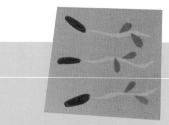

alfalfa sprouts

Alfalfa is not a bean but a tiny grain, although it can be soaked in the same way as beans to make a pleasant-tasting, nutty sprout that is rich in protein and nutrients. Alfalfa sprouts contain calcium, zinc, iron, potassium and magnesium, and the eight essential amino acids. They are useful for the treatment of fatigue, colds, stomach ulcers and urinary problems, as well as helping to reduce plaque formation in the arteries.

• High-energy fruit like figs, bananas, custard apple and lychees.

• Grated coconut.

• Milk shakes with fresh cream and fruits to camouflage the cream. Add crushed almonds, hazelnuts or cashew nuts to add flavour and texture to the shake.

If you manage to get them to eat eggs too, you will have won a great battle.

Instead of water, use a nutritious home-made stock to cook rice and pulses, or as a base for vegetable soup. Make the stock from meat bones or a chicken or poussin carcass (see page 166), but remove or mask the meaty smell as much as possible. Much of this comes from the skin and fat, so skin poultry before cooking and carefully remove excess fat from the stock (either soak up with overdone dry toast or leave to cool and lift off the solidified fat from the surface). Garlic, ginger, a pinch of nutmeg, saffron, bay leaves or cardamom will all help disguise the smell further.

There are many varieties of protein powders for vegetarians available in healthfood shops. A couple of scoops in milk, water or juice will help to keep the protein intake stable. This may go down best after a vigorous work-out, in order 'to replenish energy'.

With psychological help there will be, hopefully, an improvement in mental state, and you can graduate to a more varied diet. Once they develop a liking for chicken or fish or meat, there is very little scope for relapse.

Constant concern about 'improving' body shape and getting rid of what is perceived as excess weight makes anorexics obsessional exercisers. You may be able to channel this into more therapeutic forms of exercise, such as dance. Highly rhythmic dance such as flamenco or Indian dance enhances the mind–body connection and is therefore useful therapy. It can lead in turn to yoga and meditation, which can help refocus body awareness.

Anorexics will often appreciate massage to relieve the discomfort from the build-up of lactic acid in the muscles brought on by heavy exercise sessions. Deep tissue massage with sweet almond oil or sesame oil helps to relax the body and induces good sleep. Take this one step further with a ghee massage.

As ghee (found in Indian grocery shops and most supermarkets) is churned and potentised butter, it is quite useful to an anorexic body – in India, babies who have a poor appetite are massaged with ghee. You can explain that it is medicinal and might prevent bone fracture and hormonal imbalance. Rub a tablespoon a day into the abdomen until it is absorbed. Some people don't like the smell, but this can be covered up with something like sweet almond oil. Over the course of a few hours the skin will absorb the ghee and the blood vessels will take up the ghee's nutrients. Ayurvedic medicated therapy oils, aromatherapy oils and oestrogen patches work on a similar principle.

bulimia

This is another psychological problem, where excessive eating is followed by vomiting (bulimia literally means eating like an ox). Again, alertness and support from parents or friends is essential – it may take quite a while for a bulimic to accept that there is a problem, and they become adept at hiding their habits.

To keep bingeing within bounds:
• Don't keep easy-to-munch snacks like sweets, ice cream, cheese, chocolates, cream, condensed milk, cakes and biscuits, or junk-food burgers, sausages etc. in the home.
• Stock up with fresh and healthy food that is used up for the main meals only.
• Encourage eating with the family, rather than out, so that foods like chips, rich or oily food and excess sugar can be avoided.
• A cup of carrot juice or barley water (see page 147) drunk before a meal helps to smooth the lining of the gut, suppressing the appetite a little.

When blood rushes to the abdomen after a meal, the brain is deprived of oxygen and glucose. The natural lethargy this causes makes bulimics more nervous, leading to anxiety and the ritualistic vomiting after meals. Help counteract this by massaging the neck and shoulders for five minutes after main meals, to encourage blood flow back to the brain. This can be almost instantly beneficial. Lying down on the floor or on a bed without a pillow for a while shortly after a meal will also help (try the Corpse Pose, see page 68). A further aid to overcoming feelings of anxiety is ten minutes of yogic breath retention (breathing in for three seconds, holding breath for six seconds and then exhaling slowly for six seconds).

Additional ways to alleviate nausea and the need to vomit are:
• Eating five small meals a day, rather than three larger ones.
• Slow eating, chewing properly and paying attention to taste. This will reduce the volume of food eaten, as the 'stomach full' message will get through from the brain before too much more has been consumed.
• No fluids for at least an hour after eating (sip water during a meal), to ease digestion.

chapter 10
adult life

Once we reach adulthood our lives take very divergent paths. Our bodies all have the same basic nutritional requirements, but the energy needs of, for instance, a bricklayer, a professional sportswoman, an office worker and a teacher are very different. An air-traffic controller has to learn to balance a sedentary job with stressful brainwork and unsocial hours, while a mother of several young children may find either the day has gone before she has had time to think about food for herself, or that she has been snacking all day as she fed the various members of her family. We also frequently forget to take account of changing our diet when our lifestyle changes. Particular landmarks are pregnancy and retiring, so these have their own chapters.

what muscles need

If you are in a highly active job, or one that puts great demands on you physically, you are going to need strength and stamina. This will come from well-developed muscles, which means protein.

what the brain needs

The brain needs protein for its initial development and growth. But, unlike, say, blood and skin, it does not renew its cells once development is complete, so an adult brain requires only oxygen and glucose, supplied by blood and the cerebral spinal fluid, and some essential elements. As regards its main source of nutrition, glucose, the brain doesn't take account of whether this is coming from protein, vegetables or fat – a brain would make a very bad dietitian.

Essential among the elements that the brain needs to function are sodium, potassium and

the high-protein diet

This kind of diet is often favoured by athletes, as well as by people who want to lose weight quickly. But does it work, and is it a good idea?

When you cut out carbohydrates and eat solely fats and protein, the fuel supply to the body is reduced drastically. In order to generate energy, the body breaks up and uses fats to produce the energy in the contrived absence of carbohydrates. That's why you lose weight.

However, using fats rather than carbohydrates to produce energy results in the release into the bloodstream of chemicals called ketones. In excess, these cause a chemical imbalance known as ketosis (a condition that also occurs in diabetics unable to metabolise carbohydrates). Left unrectified, ketosis can lead eventually to coma and death.

High muscle power requires higher protein intake, but it is also vital to maintain a balance in your diet. If you are in serious athletic training, follow the advice of a qualified nutritionist who specialises in sports training.

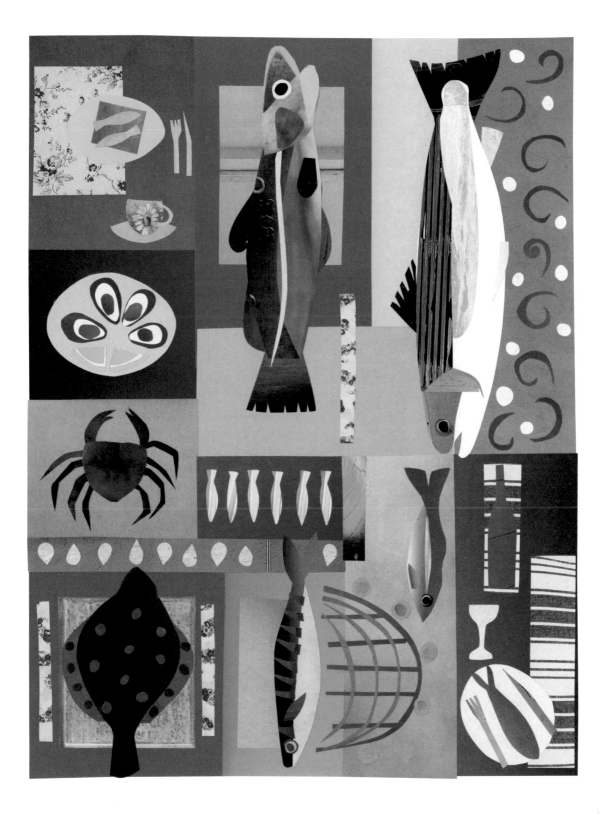

phosphorus. Fish is a good source of potassium and phosphorus (see illustration page 91), hence the belief that fish is good for the brain and fish eaters are intelligent. Nerve cells cannot function without sodium and potassium, which control the electrical properties of membranes. Just as in school, when you put metal plates in a solution of salt and water and measure the volts of electricity across the plates, so the sodium and potassium in the body need water to generate the electrical charges that 'fire' our brain. Thus water is also basic to the nervous system. We can also feel the effect of sodium on our moods: too much and we become tense, while too little makes us feel weak and low.

Nobody is all brains or all brawn. Even if you are sitting at a desk all day your posture muscles are at work and, hopefully, you are exercising to counteract the effects of a sedentary job. But in principle, those who do physical work need more protein, to give their muscles energy and to repair the wear and tear, while those who do mental work need more carbohydrates, to be converted into glucose for the brain.

breakfast

If you haven't overeaten the previous night, the digestive system should have finished its work before you went to sleep, so ideally you will be taking breakfast on an empty stomach. The job of this first meal, therefore, is to get the digestive system going again and to provide you with the right amount of energy for the work you are going to do during the morning.

As soon as you wake up drink a glass or two of warm water. This helps bowel movements. It also swills out excess acid and undigested food particles that might have been in the stomach for some time. Warm water will also reduce any tendency to eat too much for breakfast, as it washes away acids, the main stimulants of appetite. A little bit of yoga exercise each morning before breakfast will make you fit for the day.

Breakfast should not be a heavy meal because you are going to be active immediately after it and remain so all morning. This is no time to become drowsy. Eating fried food for breakfast puts a lot of stress on the stomach. You have starved overnight and need to start the day with something that will give you instant energy and is quickly digested. A plate of, say, bacon, sausages, hash browns and sautéed mushrooms will remain in the stomach, diverting energy from other activities and creating a heavy feeling that will make you disinclined to face the morning with verve and enthusiasm. Save big cooked breakfasts to have as relaxed brunches at the weekend.

As soon as you start eating, the liver will be stimulated to release some of its stored glycogen, providing instant energy. This will need to be replaced by easily digested carbohydrates. You also need some fibre to get your intestines working again and, to sustain your energy for the morning, some easily digestible protein.

For simple carbohydrates and fibre have:
• Fruit.
Ideal breakfast fruits are papaya, grapes, apples and pears. Papaya helps with bowel movements and is useful to the liver, particularly if you have had some alcohol the night before.

For complex carbohydrates have:
• Cereal or porridge.
• Soda bread, rye biscuits or rice cakes.
Soak oatmeal or cracked wheat for half-an-hour and then add some milk (or soya milk or water) and boil, stirring well until soft and homogeneous. For added energy add honey, soaked raisins and a chopped banana.

For protein have:
• Milk (if not lactose intolerant).
• Cottage cheese or yoghurt.
• Eggs.
These will also contribute to the supply of vitamins and minerals you need on a continuing basis. For extra protein, try:
• Bean sprouts a couple of times a week. Sprout

kick-start your day the caffeine-free way

Many people believe they can't function properly until they've had a fix of caffeine first thing in the morning. They think it wakes them up. And in a way it's true. It tenses up muscles, increases the heart rate, constricts blood vessels, and as a result puts the body into a heightened state of alertness. In other words, caffeine mimics tension or stress. The so-called 'kick' is the sensation of the body tensing itself for 'fight or flight'.

Drinking coffee day in and day out has a cumulative effect. The coffee of yesterday still acts today, and so you become very tense. Stop the 'fix' and you may experience withdrawal symptoms such as headaches and bad moods. Anything that produces such a withdrawal syndrome must be working on the nervous system and the physiology of the body. Ultimately caffeine is a drug and should be used cautiously, especially if you are under pressure, because it has the same effect as stress on the body, redoubling the tension.

So, how can you overcome cranky morning tiredness without resorting to caffeine? It is internal problems, joint stiffness, poor health and poor circulation that make you feel tired. Sinuses blocked with mucus, dehydration and mild hangovers all contribute to feeling below par, and overriding the symptoms with a cup of coffee is not the answer. Look instead to sensible food planning together with exercise and relaxation techniques. Herbal teas, instead of coffee, are an antidote to stress. For more on delicious caffeine-free drinks see pages 113 and 147.

your own (see page 52) and eat them sprinkled with a little salt and a few drops of lemon juice.
• A handful of almonds soaked for 24 hours and their skins removed. These are a good source of natural protein for vegans.

If your work is highly physical in the afternoon as well as the morning, breakfast has to be light but substantial, the main meal. You will need to have lunch (see pages 94–6) but your main energy for the day will come from breakfast.

Follow, say 15 to 20 minutes later, with a cup of tea. This has a certain amount of caffeine, but if taken weak is a good start to the day. If you have eaten live yoghurt, delay having a hot drink for a couple of hours, as neither hot liquid nor tannin is ideal for the bacteria.

have a break

The tea break is a long-standing tradition. The body needs a rest. A break from mental work can be a short walk or even just 'switching off' for a little while, but physical work needs physical rest: fatigue is generally muscular so you should rest periodically, sitting down.

If your muscles are tired you may feel you need an energy boost, but sweet tea or sugary cold drinks and a doughnut or slice of cake are the wrong things to have. They encourage your body to produce more lactic acid instead of drawing on your reserves.

A good breakfast based on proteins and complex carbohydrates will give you the stores of energy you need during a day's work. Instead of spending half a break organising the food and drink, just sit and give your body what it needs: a rest. Drink some water or weak, mildly sweetened tea or herbal tea to keep up your fluid intake. Sugar will activate the digestive system and drain your energies even further. You must feed on the energy reserves that your body has stored. If you take in sugary snacks every time you rest, your body has no need to draw on its reserves and they will turn to fat. You will find you put on weight even though you are doing a lot of hard physical work. In addition, if you have a problem with candida or gut yeast (see pages 184–5), the sugar will be converted to toxic alcohols and you will feel 'heady' and very tired an hour later.

lunch

After a morning's work, whether it's active physically or mentally or both, your body will need a rest and more fuel. For some people lunch is a heavy four-course meal with wine, while for many it is no more than a moment snatched for a sandwich or even skipped altogether. According to our biorhythms, this is when we should be eating our main meal of the day, when the digestive system is at its most active.

lunch on the run

Sandwiches may seem like the ideal solution, especially if you are working in the middle of a town and there is a sandwich shop on every corner; some companies will even deliver them to your desk. But, because of its yeast content, bread is not my recommendation. Similarly, the yeast in such lunchtime fare as pizzas and beer makes these an unfavourable choice. Many people notice that an hour or so after eating something yeasty they feel very drowsy and lightheaded, sometimes unbearably so. This is caused by the fermenting that the yeast causes in the gut and the resulting rise in blood alcohol levels. (See pages 44–5 for more on the action of yeast in the gut.)

A healthier choice is a jacket potato (see illustration below), with a topping of cottage cheese, scrambled eggs, tuna, sardines, prawn cocktail, hummus or baked beans. Salad, coleslaw

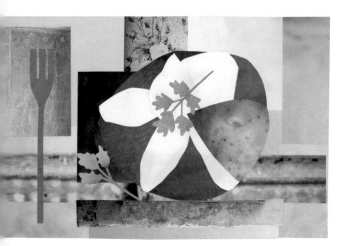

or avocados make good accompaniments. If you are at home, you can create all sorts of great toppings, from spicy mince (the mince on offer in a fast food or sandwich emporium is unlikely to be high quality) to guacamole. If you have used up a lot of energy, have two potatoes with different toppings and supplement them with some carrots and fruit.

Many sandwich shops and the like are also branching out from the basic filling between two slices of bread. Look out for stuffed tortilla wraps, trays of Japanese-style snacks and rice- or noodle-based salads.

Other alternatives to sandwiches that are available from high-street outlets include:
• Scotch eggs.
• Falafel and hummus.
• Ready-cooked chicken pieces.
• Soup (leek and potato, sweetcorn, carrot or Scotch broth are particularly filling).

One of the reasons sandwiches are such an easy option is that the ingredients are almost always to hand. So make sure you have alternatives available just as easily. Here are some suggestions:
• Ready-washed salad.
• Raw vegetables ready to munch on: carrots, celery, cucumber, spring onions, sweet peppers, cherry or small plum tomatoes.
• Dips like hummus, salsa or spicy bean.
• Bean sprouts.
• Pots of yoghurt.
• Cottage cheese.
• Tortilla wraps.
• Non-yeast breads, like soda bread, or breads lower in yeast, like pitta.
• Fruit.

Whether you are at home or going out to work, it will take but a moment to concoct a good lunch from these basics. Supplement them with yesterday's leftovers, such as cold roast chicken or slices of roast beef. For more ideas, see school lunches (pages 78–9).

So many people are in a constant rush and eat on the move. If you walk around eating a sandwich, or worse still a hamburger, you are

quick lunches

You won't want to keep leftovers for any length of time, but if they are covered or wrapped and stored in a cool place they will prove invaluable when you are looking for a quick lunch the next day. You can even cook extra on purpose, to save time the following day. Rice makes a good salad base, as do new potatoes and pulses such as chickpeas or black-eyed beans. Pulses can also be blended to a purée with garlic and spices to make an excellent home-made dip, or have with salad in a tortilla wrap.

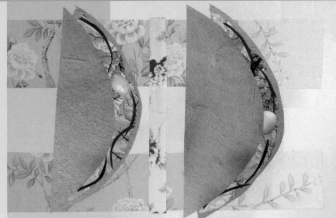

dividing your energy, putting unnecessary strains on other systems and focusing on neither. Sitting at a desk and working as you eat is just as bad. Because you are not paying attention to your food you will be inclined to gulp it instead of chewing properly. If you eat quickly you are likely to eat more than you need, and when you eat without noticing you will later miss that sense of satisfaction at having enjoyed your food, and feel the need for more food, not because you are hungry, but because you want the sensation of eating.

business lunches

The concept of the business lunch is a bizarre notion, almost as absurd as the business breakfast. Both evolved for two reasons: to squeeze extra working time into the day and to soften up the ground on which proposals can be discussed and agreements made.

Business is best done during business hours. Allowing it to invade lunchtime denies you what you need in the middle of the day: a chance to refuel your body and rest your brain. In a business lunch you are focusing on conversation and not taste. However apparently relaxed the setting, there is a war of nerves being played across the table.

If you are able to, get the business out of the way before you eat, and then concentrate on the meal separately. An alternative is to leave it until just after lunch, but your brain will be less alert then, and the anticipation of negotiations may make you tense during the meal.

There is an important difference between talking while you are actually eating and talking while you are digesting. The latter is perfectly all right, but the former encourages you to gulp your food. You want to empty your mouth as quickly as possible, which means you don't savour the food, you don't chew properly and you swallow air as you gulp. All this will play havoc with your digestion. To make matters worse, you have not even enjoyed the food because your attention has been elsewhere – most people do not remember what they have eaten at a business meal.

If you are faced with no alternative but to discuss key issues as you eat, here are some ways to minimise the harm it does.
• Because business lunches are much about creating an impression, it is all too easy to eat and drink more than you intend. Remind yourself of this before you meet, to guard yourself against saying yes for the sake of appearances or to please your host or guest.
• For a starter, choose either soup or a salad, something that you cannot swallow down without noticing. Soup will force you to pause as you

concentrate on not spilling the spoonful, allowing you to pay attention for a while on what you are eating; it is also easy to digest. A salad needs to be chewed. Not only will you be able to digest well-chewed food more easily, but having to chew each mouthful draws your attention to what you are eating and keeps you alert.

• Similarly, for the main course, choose something that will demand your attention: fish or meat that needs to be cut off the bone, vegetables like asparagus or broccoli that you can't just scoop up unthinkingly.

• Get into a rhythm of chew and listen, stop and talk. Give the other person a chance to do the same. Set a calm pace and you have a better chance of understanding the business under discussion. If others at the table are at times in a position to be able to talk when you can't, so be it. Their health is their affair, and there is a lot to be said for listening more than you talk.

• Choose only a very light dessert or none at all – you are unlikely still to be hungry. If the lunch is a drawn-out affair, with long pauses between courses, then your digestion will have had sufficient time to accommodate a dessert. Biscuits and cheese are not a bad choice because they amount only to a small portion, for the taste. Avoid fungal cheeses such as blue-veined and soft, rinded cheeses.

• Business lunches are generally less boozy affairs than they used to be, but there may be drinks beforehand and wine with the meal. The message here – as always – is moderation. Too much alcohol, or alcohol on an empty stomach, will start to take effect towards the end of the meal, blunting your mind just when you may need to be at your sharpest for the concluding part of the business. Have a soft drink before the meal and enjoy a glass of wine at the table. Taking the wine with food will slow down the absorption time of the alcohol. And drink your wine in sips. It will give you more pleasure and affect your alertness less. If you are lunching out several times a week you may find it preferable to avoid alcoholic drinks altogether – socially an increasingly acceptable option.

If full-blown business lunches or dinners are a regular feature of your life you may feel you can survive, even thrive, on such a regime, but it will take its toll sooner or later. Don't wait until plumpness turns into obesity, or your heart or liver gives up in protest. Mitigate the effects now: keep your other meals very simple; become a weekend vegetarian; do a one-day full fast (see page 57); and treat your digestion to food that is easy to deal with, such as purées and soft, bland food.

digestion time

Whatever you have eaten, within the hour all this digestive activity diverts blood to the abdomen at the expense of other parts of the body and makes you feel drowsy. This is natural. If you put energetic demands on your body at this time, while it is trying to do its principal digestion of the day, it does you no good. You should not do anything too energetic (sport or heavy exercise, have sex, carry heavy things) on a full stomach. Either your digestion is impeded by trying to do heavy work, especially physical work, or your energy will be channelled into digesting all your food and you will have much less energy for other functions. In an office, if you get straight back to work after a full meal, the natural dip in the blood circulation makes you irritable, even angry, impairs your performance and you feel stressed.

If at all possible, try to allow yourself a rest after lunch. Even half an hour can be a great help – the siesta is sensible, not lazy! If you cannot, and you have to work right through the day without a proper break, then it is not practical to have so much for lunch. Stick to something very light (soup with no bread, salad or just fruit).

the evening meal

If you have eaten well for breakfast and lunch, there is no need for dinner to be a heavy meal. However, most people in today's world have made dinner the main meal. It is a time to relax after a hard day's work and there is a better chance of savouring your food than during a truncated break

time for a siesta

Digestion diverts blood and energy to the stomach, giving you initially less energy to do other things. Relieving your muscles of the work of keeping you balanced and upright gives the stomach a chance to do its job better.

My mother used to say: 'After lunch, lie five minutes on the left side, ten minutes on the right.' This is not just a fanciful old saying: lying on the left side helps acid secretion and the churning of food, while lying on the right helps enzyme secretion. So doing this encourages the stomach juices to absorb food and begin the digestion process.

Resting does not necessarily have to be in the horizontal position, as the stomach's initial churning is not reliant on gravity. But lying down will encourage you to feel sleepy, and accepting this rest as mental as well as physical will give your brain a chance to rest too.

the practice

It would be enormously beneficial if more places of work provided quiet rooms for staff after lunch. Coffee rooms and staff rooms could be used in this way, but are usually full of chatter and noise.

Take advantage of a nearby park and in good weather lie on the grass or sit on a bench quietly for 15–20 minutes. This sort of change of scene, away from distractions such as telephones or demands on your time from colleagues, customers or charges, is hugely beneficial.

If you can't get out, see if you can find a quiet room or area and try this short version of yoga sleep:

1 Rest your head on a table, cushioned on your folded arms.

2 Close your eyes and breathe gently.

3 Focus your concentration on your neck. Imagine it relaxing, the tension going out of it. Do the same for your upper back and shoulders, mid-back, lower back, buttocks, thighs, calves, ankles and toes, in that order.

4 Repeat this seven times. Then switch your thought to your shoulders, arms, wrists, hands and fingers, in that order. Again, repeat seven times.

5 Relax your eyelids, eye muscles, temples, jaw and cheeks. Imagine that your body feels relaxed and heavy. Picture your muscles expanding and allowing fresh blood into them.

6 Stay in this state for 10–15 minutes and you will feel refreshed and ready to face the afternoon.

You can practise this even if your only source of retreat is your desk or a table in an unobtrusive corner. For a fuller version of yoga sleep see page 69.

Alternatively, massage your neck and shoulders using your thumbs and fingers. Squeeze the neck and shoulder muscles and then let go. Fresh blood will rush in when you release the pressure and remove the lactic acid which is the main cause of pain and those sore knots or lumps of tightened muscles. Repeat several times.

Do head rolls. Look over your left and right shoulders alternately, stretching the muscles. Grab your left shoulder with your right hand, keeping your shoulder straight, then pull your left shoulder forward while turning your head to look over your left shoulder. Do the same thing on the right side. This will stretch and release the neck muscles.

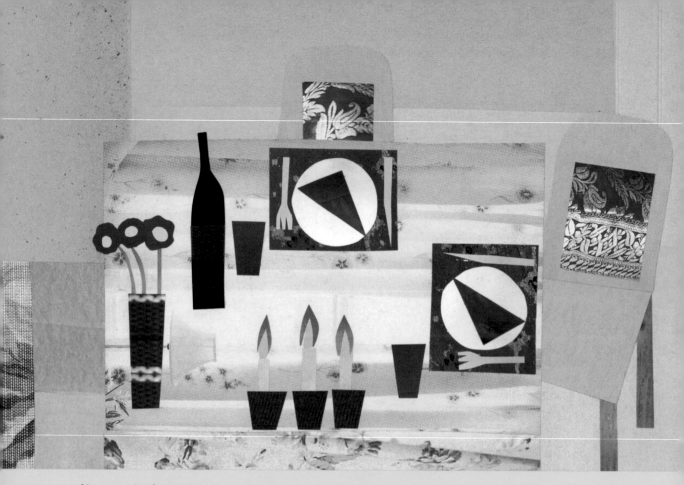

dinner à deux

The table is set, the candles are lit, romantic music plays softly. First, a relaxing apéritif, or two. Or perhaps, to keep the atmosphere lighthearted to begin with, a couple of fun cocktails. Then champagne – of course. Need to impress with the food, so there's lobster thermidor to start, then beef Wellington, and a luscious creamy confection for dessert. The wine's good too, and plenty of it. A fine choice of cheese to finish (the runny blue French one looks particularly ripe), perfect with a glass of that vintage port you've been saving. And now for that long-awaited romantic end to the evening – but your partner's fallen asleep and your stomach's really not feeling too good at all… What a shame.

Tempting though they may be, rich, creamy dishes, and too much food and alcohol, spell disaster. A romantic dinner should be tasty but not heavy to digest – a meal that gives your stomach too much work to do will leave you no energy for anything else.

Avoid fried or oily food, and plan a menu around just one protein-rich dish – don't choose fish for a starter and then have meat for the main course, for instance. Spices like paprika, garlic, ginger, saffron and mustard help tone up the body. (And, should you wish to include soft-boiled eggs in the meal, they help men to produce more sperm and the protein will refuel the body later.) Save dessert for after an intimate time, when you will appreciate it most.

Omar Khayyám, the Persian poet, enjoyed the company of his love with wine – but getting drunk, or getting your partner drunk, is completely the wrong thing to do. Champagne is celebratory, but on an empty stomach its bubbles hasten the effect of alcohol. A moderate amount of alcohol, savoured slowly, adds to the relaxed, intimate atmosphere, but the full effect of drinking too much will only hit you an hour or two later – alcohol may lower inhibitions but it also impairs sexual performance.

in the middle of the day. It is also often the only time families can sit down and enjoy a meal together. The body has also adapted to this regime over the years, but it is still important to remember that whatever you eat now should be digested before you go to bed. (Of course, if you are working night shifts, eating before going to work is perfectly all right, as your body will have reversed its cycle. In this case it's your last meal before you go to bed, which may be at breakfast time, that should not be too heavy.)

The main problem is that many people fit the requirements of their body around their lifestyle rather than vice versa. Trying to fit in a non-stop day, then a full heavy evening meal (to make up for the food you haven't had time to eat earlier in the day), digestion time, a social life and a reasonable length of sleep at night just doesn't work, so something has to give and it's usually the digestion time. Give a little time and thought to how you structure the end of your day, and how it could be made better.

If you have a siesta after lunch this will enable you to go to bed a little later, giving your digestion time to do its work properly. If you go out dancing, walking, doing some yoga stretches, and delay bed-time to allow the food to settle down, then a full meal should not be problematic. Without these compensations, be prepared to suffer from digestive problems. The body cannot be made to digest heavy foods at night and carry out necessary repair work such as synthesising blood enzymes and working lactic acid from muscles over-used during the day. All these need energy, but the body can't do too many things with limited energy.

I advise some exercise after an evening meal, to encourage the digestive system into action, and I am often asked whether making love would be a good form of exercise – perhaps the combination of the relaxation that a little alcohol brings and the idea of combining going to bed and exercising makes this seem the perfect answer! But no, don't have sex soon after a heavy meal – it can be much more strenuous than the gentle stroll I advocate. Allow two or three hours to lapse. (The ideal time

light suppers

If you are late for dinner and have to go to bed soon after, you need something quick that is easily digested. Mashing or puréeing food gives the stomach less work to do.

• Boil a couple of eggs. Peel and mash them with a fork, add a little butter or olive oil, black pepper and salt to taste. Spread on a slice of toasted soda bread or crispbread.

• Avocados are light but nutritious, and fill a hungry hole very well. Mash one up with olive oil, a few drops of lemon, and salt and black pepper to taste.

• Fruit digests easily; accompany it with some roasted peanuts or cashews (chew them well to save your stomach the effort) and drink water.

• A cup of chamomile tea before bedtime is a good relaxant.

• Dates, figs, raisins, peanuts, cashew nuts or pecan nuts.

to have sex is actually early in the morning, when you are rested physically and mentally, and the sensory organs and erogenous zones are more sensitive but less tense.)

exercise and sport

The best time for energetic physical exercise is in the morning, before breakfast. Many people play sports after lunch. It is quite wrong. If the afternoon is your only opportunity for sports or exercise, make sure you don't have a heavy lunch that will take a long time to digest, and wait for at least two hours after your meal.

Evening is not the best time, either. A walk after dinner is helpful to get the digestion moving, but fit in anything like squash, running or a work-out class before you eat (while making sure this doesn't delay your evening meal too long). If your routine means you can only exercise later in the evening, then arrange things so that your main meal is in the middle of the day. If supper is light, then lunch or breakfast has to be substantial.

food on the move

'A traveller has to do without so many things which he is accustomed to (while he is in his home town) and so has to face hardships and illness. He must, therefore, take care of the matters concerning his body so that he might be safe from many diseases. He should pay his utmost attention to matters of diet and causes of fatigue.' Avicenna (980–1037)

Travel today is unimaginably different from the journeys Avicenna had in mind when he wrote this in his Canon a thousand years ago, but travelling still puts a great strain on the body. People still get fatigued and suffer tummy upsets, colds and coughs. Mostly, blame is put on the atmosphere in the aircraft, the local water or unhygienically prepared food. Any form of long-distance travel can upset our digestion and sleep, but it is during and after long-haul flights that people are most likely to feel unwell: the faster the journey, the greater the degree of adaptation required.

Crossing many time zones in a short period of time takes you into a topsy-turvy world where your biological clock and the actual time are separated – your body may be telling you it is night, and time to sleep, but the local clocks are saying it is lunchtime. Sleep, appetite, bodily functions and energy levels go haywire. After a long flight your digestive system functions badly, and any food, however well it is prepared and cooked, can cause bloating, diarrhoea or constipation. More often than not, these tummy upsets are not bacterial dysentery, food poisoning or 'dodgy water', but simply the body's reaction to travelling and eating different types of food. Such troubles will persist until your body has adapted. Travelling continually from one place to another has the worst effect, because the body simply doesn't get a chance to adapt.

In order to help your body adapt as quickly as possible, you need to avoid overworking your digestive system and build up and conserve your energy.

food and drink

During a long-haul flight, and for a day or two beforehand:

• Avoid alcohol, coffee, fizzy drinks, excess salt, excess citrus fruits, smoking, very spicy food or meals rich in butter, cheese, oil or cream.
• Eat vegetables, fruit and carbohydrates like rice and pasta, or perhaps some fish or chicken, but avoid hard-to-digest food like red meat.
• Drink at least 2 litres of water a day.
• Drink carrot, apple and ginger juice.
• Drink two or three cups a day of ginseng tea – ginseng is a good adaptogen.

The simpler the food on a journey, the better. Avicenna put great emphasis on drinking water. The digestive system becomes sluggish on a long journey, and water helps to wash out any putrefaction in the system caused by 'stalled' food. This slowing down of the digestion is why during and after travelling faeces and urine smell strong.

When you arrive, keep to this regime if you are on a short trip. With your body not adjusted to the new time zone, your appetite will generally be low at 'new' mealtimes, and no appetite means that the body is not geared up to receive food in quantity. Forcing food on your system at what it perceives is the wrong time is perhaps a contributing factor to travel-related digestive problems.

For longer stays, introduce new foods and new times gradually. To help your biological clock retune itself, eat dates or something sweet when you feel hungry in your 'old', biological time and eat meals at the new, local times (heavier lunch and lighter dinner if possible). If you can, eat familiar food to begin with, slowly introducing local foods. This will help the body to adjust. Drink herbal teas and juices in the first couple of days, introducing local waters slowly.

energy

To revive and refresh ourselves, we need to sleep. Jet lag throws our bodies into confusion as the secretions of melatonin, the hormone that controls sleep, and adrenaline, which regulates wakefulness,

rhubarb

The most important therapeutic property of rhubarb is that it can help to treat common menstrual and menopausal problems, such as hot flushes. It is also an effective laxative. Rhubarb's sour taste is due to its concentration of vitamin C, but adding a lot of sugar is not advisable as this affects its therapeutic quality – sweeten it instead with sweet cicely. Rhubarb contains potassium, iron and calcium, but it also contains oxalic acid, which inhibits the metabolism of iron and calcium.

are out of kilter. The greater your reserves of energy, the sooner these two hormones will come back into harmony once again.

Before travelling, light exercise, massage and moderate, untaxing meals will help build up your energy. Continue this regime on arrival, but refrain from exercise as your body is depleted of energy – it needs more rest than exercise. Take short naps (timetable permitting) to avoid drowsiness, and treat yourself to massage and yoga stretches to help renew your energy.

the difference between men and women

Just as children, teenagers, adults and the elderly should all eat differently, there are some significant differences in dietary needs between men and women, however hard people try to ignore them. The sexes are physically different, their hormones are different, so naturally there are nutritional differences too. When planning what to eat and when, women should take into account their menstrual cycle or the onset of the menopause (see pages 186–8).

Diet can have a noticeable effect on libido for both men and women. Buddhist monks generally have a simple, bland vegetarian diet, designed to decrease libido – the smaller and simpler the meal, the lower the libido.

Libido can really go up if you have a rich diet, high in protein. Vegetarian protein like soaked almonds and pistachios, milk, cottage cheese etc. are also useful. (If, however, there is no sexual outlet for this raised libido, the body's desire will drop again after about forty days.) If sexual demand is lower, men and women should eat less protein and avoid heavy foods like butter, cheese and cream as this may excite them more.

A man can provide a fillip to his libido with an egg nog about 24–48 hours beforehand. Whisk a raw egg into creamy warm milk and drink it. Be very sure the source of the egg is reliable – free-range is no guarantee and salmonella is no libido-raiser. This is a natural aphrodisiac and seems to have powerful spermatogenetic powers.

xeno-oestrogens

Oestrogen is a female hormone involved in sexual development. In recent years there has been increasing evidence that pollutants in the food chain include xeno-oestrogens, which mimic the role and nature of oestrogen. These come from a variety of sources, including leaching from some types of plastic packaging and contaminated river water, affecting fish.

An overabundance of oestrogen or oestrogen-like chemicals affects both men and women. In women oestrogen works in tandem with another hormone, progesterone, but there is a concern that an imbalance in the levels of the two hormones may contribute to breast and ovarian cancers. In men, xeno-oestrogens may play a part in falling sperm counts. There is much research still to be done in this field, but such fears only strengthen the argument for eating fresh food raised in an environmentally friendly way.

chapter 11
starting a family

Women need to take particular care of their diet and lifestyle during and after pregnancy. Pregnancy is not an illness, but it does put enormous stress on the body: hormonal changes, the physical weight of the growing baby, the need to supply the baby with adequate nutrition (eating for two doesn't mean eating twice as much but it does need to be taken seriously), the psychological adaptation to becoming a mother. What you eat just before, during and after pregnancy will affect both your own health and your baby's, now and in the future.

preparing for pregnancy

If you are planning to have a baby, it makes sense to get your body into good condition beforehand. By this I do not mean doubling your exercise routine or going on a diet – in fact being underweight will not help conception at all and, unless you are already too heavy (see pages 126–8), putting on a little weight is perfectly all right.

Ensure the food you are eating is very nutritious and providing a good balance of protein, complex carbohydrates and fat (see Chapter 1). In addition:
• Include plenty of foods rich in folic acid: lentils and pulses, kale, broccoli and other dark green vegetables, and nuts are all good sources (see illustration opposite). Folic acid is instrumental in the formation of DNA and in cell reproduction, and the usual advice is for women to take double the usual recommended amount of folic acid for several weeks before and after conception, so you may take a supplement as well.
• Avoid raw eggs and unpasteurised dairy products.
• Have a complete ban throughout your pregnancy on alcohol and smoking. Alcohol can threaten or damage the foetus and is best avoided altogether. These, as well as coffee and high-caffeine energy drinks, affect the hormones and the way they function.
• Eat pomegranates, as they help synthesise blood.

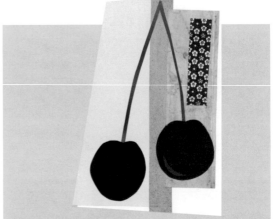

cherries

Cherries are often recommended to women during pregnancy and after childbirth. They contain useful amounts of vitamin C, zinc and iodine (which is helpful in the treatment of thyroid malfunction). Their ability to dilate the bronchial tract mean they give relief from an asthma attack, and are used to ease coughs and bronchitis. Cherry brandy is a powerful tonic used for low blood pressure and energy. Brandy is a strong alcohol, however, so it should not be consumed in large quantities.

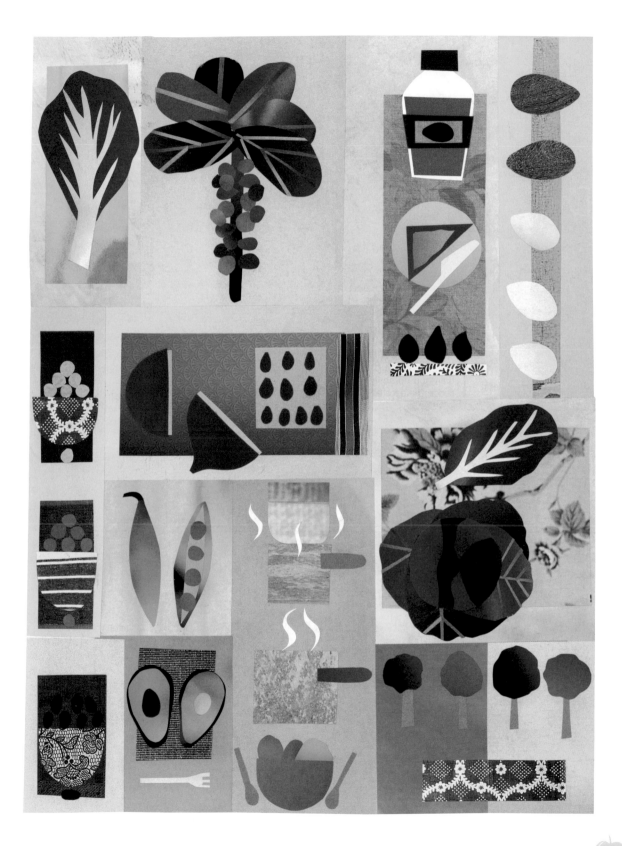

Continue to follow these guidelines throughout your pregnancy.

Now is a good time to begin a yoga or gentle exercise or meditation class, so that it has become a habit when you most need it later.

The stages of pregnancy divide themselves quite neatly into three three-month segments, called trimesters.

the first trimester

The symptom most associated with the early stage of pregnancy is morning sickness. This happens (and not necessarily in the morning) because of the trauma of your body having to adjust to such a new situation. As well as hormonal changes, it has detected a foreign body – the embryo, with genes and proteins from the father – which it is programmed to reject. The fertilised egg grows very rapidly, demanding fluids and nutrition via the placenta, drawing on the mother's nutrient supply. In response the mother's body tries to upset the food intake, and the result is an aversion to food, with nausea sometimes at even the sight or thought of it. Yet the mother's body of course still cries out for food.

Recognising what is causing this conflict is a help. It is important that you do not starve yourself (and, critically, your baby) of vital nutrition. Try several very small meals a day, rather than the regular breakfast, lunch and dinner. You may find that some times of the day are better for eating than others – listen to your body rather than watching the clock.

Protein is the building block of all growth in the body. Foetal growth is very rapid and the supply of protein has to be constant, but pregnant women sometimes find they have an aversion to eggs, fish, beef, lamb and so on, usually because their distinctive smells trigger nausea. Camouflages like garlic or other strong-smelling herbs may be intolerable themselves, especially in the first trimester. Instead, try using vegetables like spinach and tomatoes to mask the smell. A Spanish omelette or an Indian masala omelette are full of

relief from morning sickness

• Sniffing a fresh green lime suppresses nausea when you feel a bout coming on. This is astonishingly effective.
• Lentil soup. Soak lentils for two hours or so, rinse thoroughly and cook to a pulp. Add salt and black pepper to taste; blend and sieve. A few drops of lemon juice will improve the taste. Drink cold, and have two or three bowls a day.
• Almond milkshake. Soak almonds for 24 hours. Peel, and grind to a paste in a food processor. Add milk, a couple of scoops of plain vanilla ice cream and blend together. This makes a refreshing and nutritious shake.
• A banana mashed with fresh cream and a little sugar or maple syrup.
• Carrot and apple juice.

vegetables. Try chicken with spinach or spit-roast chicken flavoured with sage, barbecue or tandoori sauce or in a light garlic and butter sauce. If even disguised animal protein is temporarily unacceptable, see page 36 for advice on rich protein sources for vegetarians and vegans.

Alleviating stress and staying relaxed also helps minimise the nausea. At bedtime or first thing in the morning massage your neck and shoulders, or, better, ask your husband or partner to do it for you. Spray lavender mist on the pillow at night to help you have a good night's sleep.

Not everyone suffers from morning sickness and, by three months, the adaptation is complete and the nausea usually goes.

dietary supplements

Nutritional requirements change surprisingly little during pregnancy as long as you are following a healthy eating regime and do not go on a slimming diet or develop an aversion to something you would normally eat. Some nutrients that mothers-to-be may feel they need more of are:

Calcium

Both mother and unborn child need plenty of calcium, but taking supplements is usually unnecessary as the body is triggered into absorbing calcium more efficiently. You should, however, do all you can to help this absorption. Diarrhoea and chronic constipation can both impair calcium and magnesium absorption, so ensure your bowels stay in good working order. A bit of sun, exposing as much skin as possible (just sitting in a sunny window if the weather is cold), will provide enough vitamin D to optimise calcium absorption.

Zinc

This trace element is included in the typical multivitamin + mineral supplements that most doctors recommend during pregnancy. It is also present in root vegetables (carrots, turnips and beetroot), spinach, broccoli, asparagus, tomatoes, apples and apricots. Unless you are deficient (perhaps you have a weak immune system resulting in frequent colds and coughs or excessive allergies during hayfever season), zinc in a separate form should not be necessary.

Iron and folic acid

These are recommended in supplement form as they are an essential part of haemoglobin or blood synthesis and are needed during pregnancy to cope with the demand for extra oxygen from the rapidly growing foetus. Good sources of iron and folic acid are: spinach, pomegranates, aubergines, red apples, red meat and 'fortified' breakfast cereals. Pulses and brassicas are also rich in folic acid.

In traditional Asian societies women don't eat ginger or papaya while they are pregnant because both these have powerful enzymes and alkaloids (so powerful they are used in tenderising meat) and are said to cause miscarriage or bleeding.

the second trimester

Once her body has accepted the new life growing inside her, a mother-to-be's appetite usually returns in full force. Sometimes it is as if the taste buds crave stimulation.

Take time to plan your life over the next few months. Your appetite is now driven by two requirements: your own and the unborn baby's. Your baby's demands will trigger appetite independently, but your own needs will depend on the life you are leading.

If you are pushing your body as hard as you

food cravings

I well remember that, in India, a tell-tale sign that a member of the family was pregnant would be her unusual food cravings, typically for sour, vinegary tastes. A mother-in-law's first indication that her daughter-in-law was pregnant might be when she caught her in the kitchen sneaking a spoonful of pickles or quietly crushing lemon leaves to smell.

Some of the food cravings by pregnant women seem like a joke: chalk, earth, coal. But they can be a useful signal that the body needs more of a certain substance. While the foetus's bones are developing, the demand for calcium shoots up. You may find yourself hankering for milk and cheese, but also bones or even chalk. Indian village women might break clay pots and chew the pieces. Not very appetising, but clay is full of calcium.

In the later stages of pregnancy the blood supply to the mother's brain may decrease as the baby's activity increases. This will signal itself in a need for glucose, resulting in a craving for anything sweet.

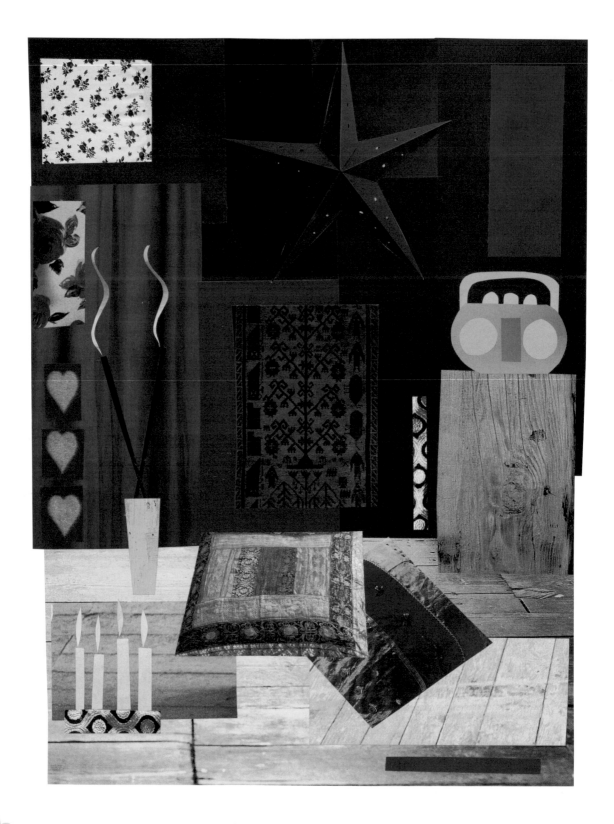

did before, your appetite will increase but your ability to burn off those calories will be less as the baby becomes more burdensome. Your body needs these reserves.

If you ignore your body's demand for extra nutrition, the baby will claim nutrients that you need and you will become run-down and overtired, perhaps anaemic. In turn this will affect the size of the baby (which your doctor will warn you about after a scan).

If you reduce your demand for energy (both physical and mental) your appetite will be lower – but if you continue to eat the same out of habit you will put on unnecessary extra weight. Women who take long pregnancy leave and sit at home often eat more out of boredom.

So, it is all a question of balance. Listen to your body: nature knows that whatever goes on in the environment of the mother affects the foetus, and during pregnancy the body becomes very sensitive.

Make resting a positive part of your day, not just a response to exhaustion. Walk regularly twice a day in the fresh air, and meditate frequently in a peaceful environment (see illustration opposite). Don't feel guilty about doing nothing. You will know already that I am a great advocate of the siesta (see page 97). This is even more important now. Go to bed early and don't force yourself to 'rise and shine' early in the morning.

the third trimester

Just as the first trimester concentrates on preserving the foetus, the third prepares for the baby's birth. By this time your hormones have adjusted, your body has regulated itself and many women are amazed and delighted to find that chronic troubles such as allergies, asthma and migraine disappear.

Make sure that you are getting enough protein. As well as being necessary to manufacture haemoglobin, proteins give strength to stretched skin and provide enzymes for body repair. A lack of protein is very unlikely if you eat fish, meat and eggs, but vegetarians should ensure they are getting sufficient through dairy products, and vegans will need to get their supply from beans (especially soya beans), nuts and pulses combined with grains. For more on protein, see pages 14 and 36.

Constipation can sometimes be a problem in the late stages of pregnancy, so eat easily digestible food and plenty of fresh fruit and insoluble fibre (from rice, beans and vegetables) to prevent this. Also drink plenty of water (2 litres a day), even though your bladder has less room to expand.

If you are eating and resting sensibly you should not be putting on excess weight, but do not consider weight or weight gain now. It is natural to put on weight. Many women remain highly concerned about their weight, and it adds an absolutely unnecessary stress. After the baby is born there is a natural tendency to lose weight if you look after yourself, and massages can be helpful then.

The main thing is rest. To work up to the last day of pregnancy is absurd. This is one of the main causes of women suffering when giving birth. So many delayed births and premature babies are as a result of the woman not being in tune with Nature, and not taking everything in moderation. My

good foods for pregnant women

- Pomegranate juice.
- Home-made shepherd's pie.
- Chicken and vegetable casserole.
- Fish or meat pie.
- Dates, figs and raisins.
- Kichri rice with yoghurt, or rice pudding, if you aren't feeling hungry.
- Carrot and apple juice.

hassle-free food

With your life turned upside down, and no routine, this is a time when it is very easy to eat badly, just when you're in particular need of nourishing food. Do all you can to have good, fast food made easy:
• A hotchpotch similar to that recommended to the elderly is often handy (see page 116). Buy chopped (fresh) vegetables from the supermarket. Dice chicken breast/salmon/tuna/swordfish steaks, stir-fry with olive oil, black pepper and salt. Eat with rice.
• Kichri rice (see page 73) is quick and nutritious.
• A roast can last several meals (encourage another member of the family to do the initial cooking). Jazz up leftovers with a quick sauce of tomato purée, a little mustard, garlic paste, salt and black pepper to taste. Simply add hot water in small amounts until you have the right consistency.

• Jacket potatoes with fillings are quick to make or easy to buy, as are tortilla wraps with stir-fried vegetables.
• Soups drunk like a hot beverage throughout the day are very useful. Home-made chicken soup (see page 166) is especially nutritious.
• Juices such as fresh carrot and apple juice with celery are more nutritious than a cup of tea or coffee. (A juicer is an invaluable piece of kitchen equipment once you are weaning your baby, so it is well worth the investment during your pregnancy.)
• Chopped cucumber mixed into live yoghurt flavoured with cumin, coriander and a little salt is a good accompaniment to a meal, and better than chutney or pickle.

advice during the third trimester is to practise relaxation and meditation, and to avoid all conflicting situations. Do gentle yoga, listen to pleasant music, enjoy warm but not hot baths. Avoid travel that puts pressure on your body: long-haul flights, rough sea journeys or long drives without an overnight stop. This is especially important if travel is likely to make you nauseous – apart from being unpleasant, being sick will deprive both of you of vital nutrition.

Those who ignore their pregnancy and carry on with life as normal usually have some complication or other. The unborn 'feels' much of the stress that the mother goes through. Why, for thousands of years, should pregnant women in traditional families in the Orient be protected if it were not a special phase in their life? You don't need scientific proof for this, just logic and instinct.

recovering from the birth

Traditionally, in India, a mother newly delivered of her child is not allowed to do anything for the first five days but rest in bed and nurse her baby. She eats only chicken soup and fruit. Only on the fifth day

does she have her first bath, and then the *dais*, the midwives, give her and the baby a massage with mustard oil, a routine that continues for 40 days.

Life being what it is, this is an unrealistic scenario for the modern mother, but recovery time and cossetting is important. It is probable you will never get all the time you ideally need (especially if your new baby has older brothers or sisters), but it is vital that you allow yourself time to recover. For nine months you have been carrying and feeding a growing baby. The birth is a shock to the system; the body needs time to heal and adjust to the new circumstances. During pregnancy your body has built up more reserves than you think and is marvellous at rebalancing itself, but it can do without unnecessary stresses at the same time. Eating heavy meals and rushing round is absolutely the wrong thing to do.

Be kind to your digestive system. For the first two days at least, stick to soups, fruit and simple things like porridge and soft-boiled eggs. Fresh chicken soup is an excellent choice, highly nutritious but easy to digest. And rest completely for at least three days.

during breastfeeding

The relationship between suckling and milk production is a very close one. A baby's instinctive suckling stimulates milk production and each new stage of development triggers the constituency of the milk to adjust to the growing baby's needs.

A new baby's high demand for nutrition is a tremendous strain and many mothers are put off breastfeeding because it is exhausting. They also feel they have lost their freedom to do anything without the baby. It's a sort of pregnancy outside the body, the baby just as dependent on its mother for food as when it was in the womb.

Because you are still needing to provide nutrition for your baby (whose requirements will increase fast now it is born) as well as yourself, keep concern about your weight to a minimum while you are breastfeeding. Once your baby is weaned there will be a natural transformation and, if you have kept eating sensibly, you should shed the extra weight. Cutting back on food while you are breastfeeding will only sap your energy.

Increase the amount of water you drink too – ten glasses or 3 litres a day would be quite reasonable. When breastfeeding starts, I recommend water flavoured with aniseed (1 tbsp of aniseed boiled up in a couple of litres of water). This helps to soothe the gut and generate milk. Don't forget that what you eat will be reflected in the milk you produce (see page 72).

The quality of milk you produce will also be affected by your state of tension – shock can even stop milk production altogether. Try to keep an afternoon siesta as part of your routine and do gentle yoga exercises daily. A neck and shoulder massage for 15 minutes twice a week helps the blood flow to the head, particularly the pituitary gland, which secretes prolactin, the milk-producing hormone. Sexual contact during the nursing period should be limited to once a week wherever possible – too much such strenuous activity adversely affects the quality of breast milk.

re-adjusting your body

Quite apart from feeding the baby, the body has a lot of re-adjusting to do in the wake of even an easy birth. Excitement over a new baby and a sense of achievement conflict with exhaustion from the delivery and feeding on demand, worries about 'not coping' and pressures of family and everyday life. Your hormones are in a state of flux. The bloom of pregnancy has been replaced by a feeling that your body is no longer your own.

Around the third day there is quite commonly a nose dive from elation to lowness, described as the 'baby blues'. Sometimes this is a dip that lasts a few days, sometimes it can descend into postnatal depression; occasionally, if not sensitively treated, it can remain for years as a black cloud. The causes of this depression, whether fleeting or serious, are a combination of factors, some psychological, some physical. Much of the psychological contributors will depend on your natural outlook on life and on the support and attitude of those around you.

On the physical side, your hormones will rebalance; they just need time. Now, more than ever, you need the energy and sense of well-being that food can provide. Unfortunately, one of the things that depression can bring on is bingeing on food. It's a very understandable vicious circle: you eat for comfort, your weight goes up, you get depressed at the shape of your body, you turn to more food for comfort ... Bingeing is the usual cause of putting on weight after pregnancy, so postnatal depression is one of the vital factors in determining weight.

Expecting to have some ups and downs can be an effective psychological buffer, and rest, relaxation and diet, once more, are vital in coping with this sense of depression. You are tired enough anyway, and everything seems worse when you are exhausted, so it is essential that you eat foods that will provide sustaining energy and that you do not expend more energy than is necessary on digesting them. That is why the hassle-free foods (opposite) make so much sense.

chapter 12
growing older

There is nothing at all we can do to halt the passing years, but we all know 70-year-olds whom we would classify as 'old' and 80-year-olds, full of life and spirit, on whom the years sit lightly. What makes the difference? Genes, of course, play a part, but the real difference is made by a positive outlook on life, regular exercise, massage (see illustration opposite) and, most importantly, a sensible diet. Illness and pain are debilitating and ageing, so doing all we can to maintain good health will transform our old age. I sometimes tell the elderly to be like a fruit on the tree, which is at its best just before it drops.

as old as you feel

We may show alarm at the first grey hair, worry over the first wrinkle, but these come long before, sometimes decades before, we can be considered 'elderly'. 'Elderly' is an ill-defined expression that has little to do with actual age, but loosely applies to an accumulation of conditions or symptoms that can apply to anyone between around 50 and 100 according to their disposition, physical and mental well-being and lifestyle. To relate how elderly someone is to actual age – as insurers, employers and the like do – is absurd. Consider a few of the common signs of ageing:

• Loss of elasticity in the skin – flaking skin, wrinkles, brown or purple patches.
• Stiffness in the joints.
• Greying hair.
• Loss of energy.
• Deterioration in strength and stamina.
• Slowing down of reflexes.
• An inability to eat certain foods any longer, or a 'delicate' digestive system.
• Reluctance to change, leading to stubbornness and falling back on familiar old habits.
• Loss of libido.
• Deterioration in eyesight.
• Some loss of memory, particularly short-term memory.

While it is unlikely that anyone will keep all these signs at bay indefinitely, some are preventable, some even reversible, and many can be delayed and limited in their effect.

irreversible trends and preventable failings

As you age, usually some time after reaching 60, physiological changes take place in the entire body and especially in the digestive system. Digestive enzyme secretion is reduced, reflecting that the body has reached a stage in life where energy requirements are likely to be less. A slower digestion is inclined to cause constipation, abdominal gas and heartburn. The colon can absorb calcium less well from hard, constipating stools, so that bones and joints in turn suffer.

Weight is another critical factor that has knock-on effects. In old age, our bodies have a tendency to gravitate towards overweight or underweight, and we do less to maintain a happy medium. Being overweight puts a strain on the heart and the lower back, hip and knee joints. Exercise will help, but when osteoarthritis (often in weight-bearing joints) sets in, the pain of moving reduces mobility, setting up a vicious circle.

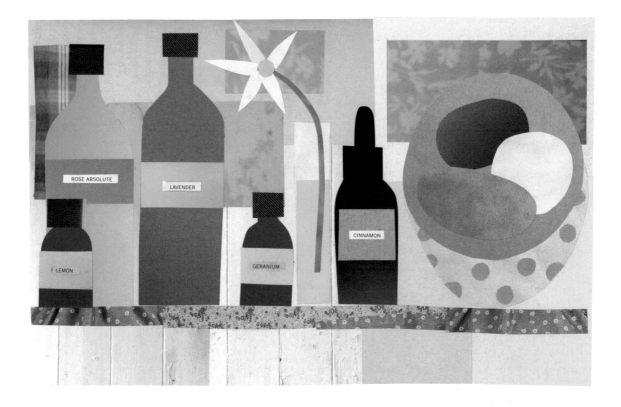

osteoporosis

This condition, also known as 'brittle bones', can occur in men as well as women, but is far more prevalent in menopausal and post-menopausal women. The cause is a loss of calcium from the bones. As osteoporosis is only partially reversible, it is important to build strong bones through childhood and early adulthood that will withstand a certain inevitable loss of calcium in later years. In later years, do not neglect your calcium intake. Good sources of calcium include:

- Fish (especially small fish where the bones get eaten as well).
- Meat.
- Dairy products.
- Dark green leafy vegetables.

Eating sufficient calcium is the first step, but it is also necessary to ensure it is absorbed properly. Our bodies do this with the help of vitamin D, which we get mostly from sunshine, supplemented by the same sorts of animal sources as calcium. So it is important to make sure you are not receiving too little vitamin D (see also page 17). There are also several things that can interfere with efficient absorption:

- Too much raw bran (which inhibits absorption).
- Problems such as chronic constipation or diarrhoea (calcium is absorbed through the colon).
- Excess coffee and tea, which encourages the excretion of calcium.

The following can also help:

- Regular weight-bearing exercises, such as walking, are very beneficial in strengthening and maintaining bones.
- Massage with sesame oil once or twice a week.
- Calcium supplements, if necessary.
- Don't smoke.
- Drink alcohol in moderation only.

Osteoporosis, poor digestion, chronic fatigue and a loss of fat reserves can make it difficult for some elderly people to maintain their optimum weight. Seriously underweight people may not be getting all the nutrition required and could suffer from mineral or vitamin deficiencies. They will also feel the cold easily, which may discourage them from going out. Sitting indoors in front of a fire all day may seem like a cosy option, but the result is likely to be stiff joints, poor circulation and boredom, all of which run counter to a healthy, happy old age.

So, many of the common complaints of the elderly – joint problems, muscular weakness, osteoporosis, digestive weakness, heart disease and diabetes – can largely be kept at bay with diet and exercise and occasional massage. A healthy lifestyle in early years will reap huge benefits in old age, but it is never too late to change.

changing requirements

Even those who have taken good care of their bodies all through their lives need to adjust to the passing years. But change becomes more difficult

anti-osteoporosis menu plan

breakfast
• Toast (use yeast-free bread) with honey, or porridge.
• Fruit: bananas, grapes, pears, apricots and peaches are all good, but avoid citrus fruits, which may cause stomach problems; their acidity also stimulates appetite.
• Once or twice a week have poached or hard-boiled eggs or cottage cheese with honey.

mid-morning
• Tea (with honey if you like) and a digestive or oat biscuit.

lunch
This should be your main meal of the day.
• For protein: fish, chicken, turkey or eggs.
• For fibre and vitamins: a variety of vegetables (well cooked) either steamed or stir-fried with a little organic sunflower oil. Red and orange vegetables such as carrots and pumpkin and dark green leaves like kale and watercress are rich in vitamin A and beta-carotene, for keeping the eyes in good shape.
• For carbohydrates: potatoes, rice or pasta.
• Live yoghurt at the end of lunch helps digestion and maintains the gut flora with useful bacteria.
   After lunch, rest or sleep for a while to aid the digestion. Lie down rather than sitting in a chair. Lying on the left side for 10–15 minutes and then on the right side for 15–30 minutes will optimise the gastric secretion and first stages of digestion.

mid-afternoon
• Tea or herbal tea (honey optional) and some oat or digestive biscuits.
   If possible, go for a walk (weather permitting) for half an hour – an hour if you can. If that is not possible, walk indoors for 15 minutes. A few yoga stretches are also good. All this aids circulation, increases metabolism and helps with the digestion and elimination of gas.

supper
One of the following, depending on how hungry you feel and what you had for lunch. This should be a smaller, lighter meal.
• Soup (mainly vegetables in chicken stock) with a couple of slices of yeast-free bread.
• Salads.
• Baked potato.
• Steamed vegetables.

bedtime
• Fruit (optional), preferably non-citrus.

a nice cup of tea

This simple, everyday beverage has a complex make-up and many variations. The name comes from the Chinese Amoy dialect, and according to legend tea was discovered in 2737 BC when a leaf fell accidentally into the Emperor's cup of hot water. He liked the flavour and aroma so much that he called it 'the drink from heaven'.

Green teas, such as Chinese and Japanese teas, are not fermented so the active ingredients are preserved. The catechins in green tea protect the walls of the body's cells and keep them healthy. Green tea aids digestion, prevents dental caries, relaxes the mind and can stop diarrhoea.

Regular tea, usually from the Indian subcontinent, is black and fermented. It tones up the body, refreshes the mind, aids digestion and can lower cholesterol. A good cup of, say, Darjeeling or Ceylon tea can bring you instant relaxation. A cup of tea after breakfast can set you up for the day, while a teaspoonful of honey in tea taken at bedtime can induce sleep. Tea contains caffeine, although less than coffee, and tannin, which can be an irritant and also interferes with the absorption of iron, so a great many cups of strong black tea is not advisable.

Herbal teas have many beneficial properties; for more information see pages 113 and 147.

---

as we age. Habits are comforting and we are inclined to cling to what we know and are used to, especially in a fast-changing world in which much of what was familiar has disappeared or moved on.

In principle, the elderly require only three-quarters or half the normal adult diet, depending on their level of activity. If you continue to eat the quantity of food you needed when you were at work all day or looking after a busy family, you are in danger of developing chronic digestive problems and putting on too much weight.

Over about the age of 70 the foods that our digestive systems find most difficult to cope with are:
• Creamy or fatty food, including cheese.
• Red meat or shellfish in quantity.
• Coffee.
• Salty foods.
• Very spicy food.
• Citrus juices.
• Excess alcohol.
• Large meals.

Perversely, these can be the very foods that hold most appeal: chocolates, cakes and biscuits are easy, moreish snacks; cream teas are a traditional treat; salt and spices add interest if the senses of taste and smell are dulled; red meat and cheese are traditional components of a meal.

Have a close look at your present diet. For one month (don't choose atypical weeks such as holiday or Christmas) keep a diary of the following:
• How many times a day you eat or snack.
• What you eat, and how much, including snacks.
• What times of the day you eat.
• What you drink and how much.
• Your bowel movements.
• Any lethargy, headaches or excessive bloating immediately after eating certain types of food.
• Any digestive problems, whether occasional or chronic.
• Whether you crave certain foods or drinks.
• What exercise you take (this covers walking round the garden or the shops as well as any more formal exercising).
• When and for how long you sleep.

After this month of monitoring you should be able to see some sort of pattern. How does it compare with the 'model day'?

This 'model day' is not a fixed prescription. Tea and biscuits mid-morning and mid-afternoon help to break up a long day, but of course they do not have to be fitted into a busy routine. We all have individual requirements and preferences, and variety and interest are important. Here are a few general guidelines to help work out a healthy, balanced eating pattern:

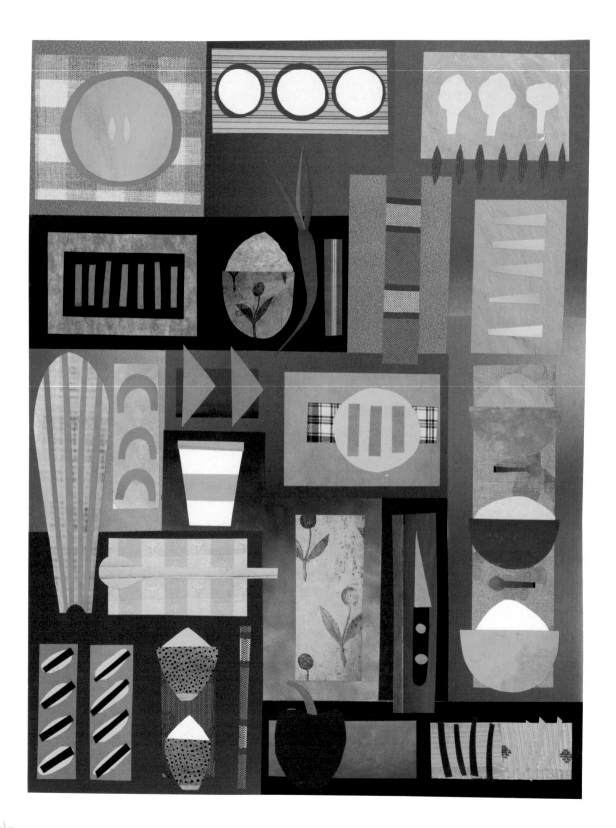

• A breakfast that is predominantly carbohydrates will be easy to digest, rather than the protein-rich breakfasts of younger people who face a day at work.
• Cereals with milk can cause a lot of wind in some people.
• If your life is largely sedentary it is best to eat two good meals a day and have a very light supper.
• White meat, fish and eggs are good sources of protein, but easier to digest than red meat.
• The insoluble fibre in vegetables helps avoid sluggish bowels, but the stalks of cauliflower, broccoli, asparagus etc. can be too fibrous and can cause abdominal gas. Just eat the heads of these vegetables.
• Try to finish supper by 7 pm. Eating late or too heavily in the evenings causes most of the digestive problems.

If gas, abdominal cramps or sinus headaches are a recurrent problem, consider your bowels! Keep a check on how often you evacuate, as constipation can lead to a number of ailments that are considered 'part of being old', but which are easily forestalled and are certainly not inevitable. See Your Health MOT (chapter 14) and the information on constipation (pages 140–44).

water
It is very tempting, if you are not very mobile, or have a weak bladder, to limit the amount of fluid you drink. However, too little water is the main cause of constipation and sluggishness, so it is important to follow the general advice and drink six to eight glasses of water per day. Some of these can be in the form of herbal or weak tea (see pages 113 and 147).

to cook or not to cook
Ideally, preparing your own fresh food is preferable to resorting to ready-made meals, takeaways and snacks. It is, however, easy to find reasons not to bother, particularly if you are not very fit and/or living alone.

'My appetite is small. It's easier just to make a sandwich or open a can when I feel peckish.'
Eating little and often is not a bad thing. It can be easier on the digestion, particularly if you separate out different types of foods (see pages 35–6). Plan ahead, so that there is something nutritious and appealing to hand when you need it.
Here are some ideas:
• Fresh fruit – reach for a pear or a handful of seedless grapes rather than the biscuit tin.
• Good-quality dips like salsas or hummus (read the labels to check what you are buying) with raw vegetables or fingers of low-yeast bread – healthier than a jam or cheese sandwich. If you enjoy cooking, make up your own dips or purées – the possibilities are endless (see illustration opposite).
• Cold meats. Buy cooked turkey by the slice at the delicatessen counter or cook a whole chicken or a double turkey breast to eat cold. Carve off slices to have with salad for an almost instant summer meal.
• Small tins of oily fish such as sardines, mackerel and tuna are useful yet healthy store cupboard staples.

'I never learnt to cook.'
Nowadays, many men are enthusiastic cooks, but that was not always so, and elderly widowers are often completely adrift in the kitchen – their wives may even have discouraged their presence in 'their domain'. Never has it been easier to learn. Don't believe that old saw about old dogs and new tricks.
Here are some ideas:
• TV cooks have taken great strides in stripping away the sham mystique of 'cuisine', and a plethora of programmes each week covers every level and type of cooking. Some will make you cringe, but there's bound to be one that hits the right note.
• A great many local authorities run adult education classes specifically for men, or geared to catering for one. A good course will also be an entertaining social occasion.
• If you rely on someone to bring in your meals, talk to them about food and ask them for advice. Begin with a small repertoire and don't feel that you will lose outside contact if you start cooking for yourself – meal providers like this recognise well the important social contact they bring.

healthy hotchpotch

Ultimately it doesn't matter to the stomach whether you eat the components of a meal separately or together. As a convenient all-in-one meal, I have designed a nutritious hotchpotch that is easy both to cook and digest. These amounts are for one person.

½ cup rice
1 chicken breast, cut into cubes
1 medium-sized potato, cut into cubes
1 medium leek, sliced into thinnish rings
1 small onion (or ½ a large onion), thinly sliced
1 carrot, sliced
½ tsp salt
½ tsp garlic purée or paste
½ tsp minced or puréed root ginger
2 bay leaves
1 cinnamon stick

1 Rinse the rice thoroughly until the rinsing water runs clear. Put it in a pan with the chicken and 2 cups of water. Bring to the boil, boil for 5 minutes, then simmer until it is softly cooked. There should be no water left by the end of the cooking time, so check from time to time that the rice is not sticking to the bottom of the pan (add a little more water if necessary).

2 While the rice is cooking, chop the vegetables and put them in a pan with 2 litres of water. Add the salt, garlic, ginger, bay leaves and cinnamon stick.

3 Add the cooked rice to the mixture and stir. Boil the entire mixture for 15 minutes.

variations:
• Use a boneless fillet of salmon instead of chicken.
• Use thyme and rosemary instead of ginger and garlic.

vegetarian hotchpotch

½ cup basmati rice
½ cup yellow lentils (moong dal)
¼ tsp turmeric
2 bay leaves
1 cinnamon stick
1 tomato, chopped
1 tsp garlic paste
a little salt
200 g frozen chopped spinach or equivalent amount of fresh spinach
1 tbsp olive oil

1 Soak the rice and lentils for about 3 hours, then rinse until the water runs clear.

2 Put the soaked rice and lentils into a pot, add 1 litre of water and the rest of the ingredients except for the spinach and oil. Boil the mixture for 30 minutes, then add the spinach and olive oil.

3 Cook everything for 10–15 minutes, stirring the mixture until it is homogeneous.

'It hardly seems worth going to all the trouble of preparing a complete meal just for one.'

If you have spent half a lifetime cooking for a family, perhaps trying to eke out a budget, it is likely you regard cooking as a chore. Time for a shift in perspective. Released from the daily grind, plan some gourmet delights for yourself. Catering for one means you only have yourself to please, and little luxuries that would be too expensive when bought for a whole family can now become affordable treats.

Here are some ideas:

• Treat yourself from time to time to a few scallops rather than a piece of cod.

• Instead of meeting friends at a café for tea or coffee, invite them to your home for a meal – sharing food is much more fun than eating alone, and however modest you are, it's a fillip to receive compliments.

• If you really have no interest in food, then pare down the effort to a minimum with one-pot hotchpotches (see opposite).

'Standing at a chopping board and hob for any length of time is too tiring.'

Cooking can certainly be exhausting if you are frail, but instead of cooking less, consider ways of making life easier.

Here are some ideas:

• There is not much more work in preparing a double or triple portion of a soup or stew. Freeze the extra in individual bags and you will have a ready-made meal on hand for minimal effort.

• Are you still cooking in the big heavy pots and pans you once used to cater for an entire family? Small pans are easier to lift, and new materials mean that lightweight no longer equates with flimsy.

• If your budget is not too tight, buy raw vegetables ready peeled and chopped. These work out more expensive and have a shorter life, but pay dividends in time and effort saved.

• Similarly, fillets of fish or chicken need no

figs

The sweet richness of figs has made them a popular fruit around the Mediterranean and the Middle East for millennia. But in cooler climates they were for a long time associated only with the pippy, pressed and dried versions that appeared around Christmas, or with syrup of figs, a traditional laxative. Fresh figs are now much more widely available, which is good news, as they are a nutritious fruit with ample fructose, minerals and trace elements. Fresh or dried, figs can boost the body's energy and therefore help in the fight against seasonal colds and sinus problems. Their anti-inflammatory properties are useful in the treatment of arthritis. Figs are high in both soluble and insoluble fibre, helping to keep the intestinal tract healthy, preventing or alleviating constipation and removing toxins from the gut.

preparation – just pop them in the oven or under the grill. Leaving them in a marinade for a while beforehand will make them even tastier without having to stand and stir a sauce.

• When relatives or friends come for a meal, ask them to chop, peel and do all the difficult and time-consuming things – they will probably be glad to feel useful (and it's usually only the washing-up that people hate doing!)

chapter 13
body types and temperaments

Not everyone has the same constitution. Some people can eat like horses and remain thin, while others seem destined to fight the fat all their lives. Some people shake off illnesses very quickly; others are laid low at the slightest hint of a germ. How we fare in life is also influenced by our temperament. People with even, nervous or fiery temperaments will react differently in the same situation or to the same ailment. Our temperaments vary according to age and circumstances, and can be modified by what we eat and how we treat our bodies. Both constitution and temperament affect your health, and may even affect whether you are regarded as healthy or not – what is a normal, expected reaction in one sort of person may be a warning sign in another. Individuals should not be measured against one standard.

types and temperaments

Centuries ago, physicians realised that people differed in certain fundamental ways, and that these differences affected their response to disease, to treatment and to food. They tried to classify these differences by referring to observable effects on the body under different conditions. For example, people who behaved and appeared as if they were being subjected to warmth or heat – that is, energetic and socially active – were referred to as being 'hot'. A silent person, wrapped up in himself and unsociable, was 'cold'. Temperamental variations like this came to be referred to as hot, cold, dry or moist.

Hippocrates put forward the theory that the body contained four fluids, which he called humours. He defined these as blood, phlegm, choler (yellow bile) and black bile. Avicenna later isolated these as being derived in digestion, and classified them as hot/moist, hot/dry, cold/moist and cold/dry. He related them to the seasons; to the elements, fire, air, earth and water (see illustration opposite); and to the stages in life in which they were dominant.

We still use words like phlegmatic and choleric to describe moods or temperaments, and talk of being 'out of humour' or 'in no humour to argue', reflecting the belief that illness occurred when any of a person's humours became imbalanced.

In ancient China and India, remarkably similar theories were developed independently. The Chinese, while identifying body fluids resembling those of Hippocrates, related constitution and temperament to the organs – again as hot, cold, moist and dry. Human characteristics, foods, even colours, were categorised into 'yin' and 'yang'. They recognised so many variations of characteristics that by the fifteenth century Teng Hong had identified 61,739 prescriptions to deal with all the permutations of disease and personality to be treated.

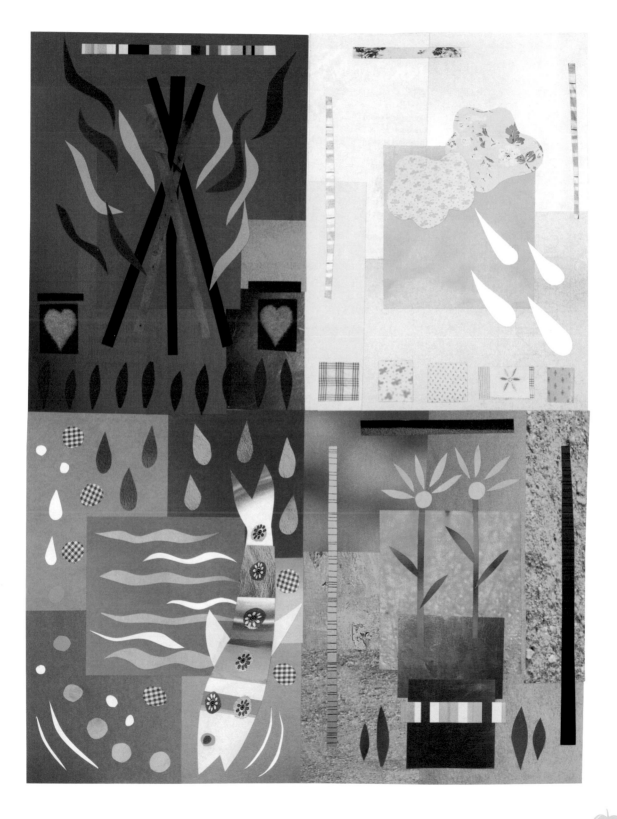

Hippocrates' four humours

blood	choler	phlegm	black bile
hot and moist	hot and dry	cold and moist	cold and dry
carrying nutrients to the heart and cells	liver residue, for digestion in the duodenum	converted into mucus, saliva and gastric fluids	affected spleen, blood and phlegm
spring	autumn	summer	winter
childhood	maturity	youth	old age
air	earth	fire	water
sanguine	**choleric**	**phlegmatic**	**bilious**

Indian traditional medicine categorised people into three doshas: Vata (active and enthusiastic, though a worrier), Pitta (sharp intellect but with a tendency to become irritable under stress) and Kapha (balanced and conservative).

In all traditions it was recognised that all the characteristics existed in everyone, and it was only the dominance of one that determined a person's personality and health requirements. Furthermore, this balance varied with age so these needs were constantly changing.

In more recent times, various philosophers and psychologists have attempted to make their own classification: Jung, for example, divided people into Extroverts and Introverts, and Pavlov categorised people as Lively, Impetuous, Calm and Weak. Others used as categories the shape of the rib cage – asthemic, normosthenic or hypersthenic; or body shapes – endomorph (rounded and soft), ectomorph (thin and angular) or mesomorph (big-boned and muscular).

We now know much more than the ancient civilisations about the body's various systems and their interdependence. We know about vitamins and antioxidants, about bacteria and viruses. And yet many of these early observations hold true, and over 20 years of experience and observation of patients have taught me that there is much to be learnt from a person's physical characteristics.

It is important for doctors to know and examine their patients when they are healthy, so that they recognise when they deviate from their individual norm. This can be a signpost to disease, which the traditional practitioner will be quick to notice. It is

the great weakness in scientific assessments of drugs or body reactions to external agents or food today that statistics are based on groups of people who are assumed equal, and take no account of different constitutions within the groups.

recognising different constitutions and temperaments

The constitution is the physical make-up of the body, including its basic functions (digestive system etc.), metabolism, speed and degree of reaction to stimuli and innate resistance to disease. Temperament is the dynamic emotional nature of a person, reflected in both physical and emotional reactions to such things as changes of environment, state of health and social situations. Temperament is a variable, contrary to constitution, which is stable or inherent. Because of this it is often difficult to measure or analyse, and described characteristics can only apply to a certain time and place; they are not immutable.

On the opposite page you'll find a guide to typical characteristics of the four basic types. I must emphasise that these are symbolic classifications offering an empirical method based on logic and not on scientific analysis, which tends to look at details rather than the overall picture. You may feel that you don't fall into any one category, but find it easier to categorise other people (and they you), and an experienced physician can do more to identify constitutional or temperamental inclinations.

To see people as one of four set types is almost as bad an over-simplification as treating everyone

the four types of constitution

	sanguine	choleric	phlegmatic	melancholic
	hot and wet (as if blood dominates)	**hot and dry** (as if bile dominates)	**cold and wet** (as if phlegm dominates)	**cold and dry** (as if black bile dominates)
skin feels	warm and moist	warm and dry	cold and moist	cold and dry
fat and flesh beneath the skin feels	firm – more flesh than fat	medium – equal flesh and fat	soft (in shorthand FFF – fat, fair and flabby)	medium – equal flesh and fat
hair	thick, straight and dark	thick, plentiful, curly and dark	scanty, straight and light coloured	thin, curly, light coloured. Prone to premature grey
skin tone*	ruddy	pale or sallow	fair	dark
body shape	broad shoulders, hips and chest, long arms, prominent joints	muscular, medium height	short, with tendency to weight gain. Men may have soft skin and enlarged breasts	medium height, thin, doesn't put on weight easily
reaction to climatic temperature	becomes restless in heat and sweats a lot	overheats in dry, desert-type weather	feels unwell in cold, wet weather, finds it hard to keep warm	worst in clear, cold weather; cold hands and feet and feels miserable
metabolism (for information on pulse rates, see pages 128–9)	good pulse rate (70–80); energetic. Good appetite and digestion with regular bowel movements	good pulse rate (70–80). Good appetite and bowel movements; high stomach acid giving, occasional indigestion and gas	slow pulse rate (60–70); feels tired sometimes; can have low blood pressure. Good appetite, but sluggish digestion and poor bowel movements	sluggish pulse (50–60); low blood pressure and often tired. Poor appetite, sluggish bowels, poor digestion
excreta	strong-smelling, dark-coloured urine, brown stools (generally)	strong-smelling, deep yellow urine. Light-coloured stools	straw-coloured urine with little smell. Light-coloured stools	infrequent dark-coloured urine Very dark stools with smell (due to putrefaction from slow digestion)
sleep and wakefulness	sound sleeper (asleep as soon as head hits pillow). Wakes early, refreshed. Has energy to work non-stop all day	often disturbed nights, but can go long time without sleep. Less tired at night, when mind very alert	likes afternoon siesta as well as a lot of sleep at night; angered if sleep is disturbed	sleeps badly (can lay awake at night worrying); feels tired during day and will catnap on journeys or in front of TVs
moods and reactions	Volatile: quick to anger but quick to cool down, without ill-feelings. Eats fast. Passionate, laughs 'from the bottom of the heart'. Makes friends easily and always cheerful. Has leadership qualities and is centre-stage in a group. Very caring. Speaks loudly. Typically optimistic	Reacts fast to emotions but cannot unwind or forget things easily. Vengeful and does not take criticism well. Listens rather than talks, but speaks thoughtfully and thinks deeply. Always calculating the next move. Often selfish and demanding	Very emotional, shy, has many fears. Hesitant to speak own mind. Difficulty in expressing deeper feelings (hides grief and nurses anger). Spiritually inclined. Great believer in destiny and luck	Pessimistic; always afraid of mishaps or disasters; smiles with great difficulty. Broods over things; yawns a lot. Inclined to dwell in the past or the future rather than live for the present. Likely to blame himself or herself for everything

*Avicenna noted that the colour of skin due to geographical location or race may camouflage the true temperament

carrots

These have been used for medicinal purposes since ancient times. The betacarotene they contain reduces the risk of heart attacks and strokes in women, while the alkaline juice is used to treat heartburn and liver problems. They also ease bowel movements and regulate gas formation in the intestines. Carrots contain a prototype of vitamin A which forms retinal, a compound that is used to synthesise visual pigments in the retina (so carrots are good for seeing, if not specifically in the dark!).

the same. We can only use this classification cautiously, as a guide, and recognise that we are each a different mix of types and have a tendency towards certain characteristics.

suiting your diet to your type

Likes or dislikes in taste, intolerances, allergies or severe aversions to certain types of food are predetermined or constitutional. Their origins can be genetic, cultural, geographical or climatic. For example, a food that is savoured by people in one part of the world may be distasteful to those in another, and may even cause nausea, diarrhoea or bloating. People from cooler zones often cannot cope with chillies, while cheese is quite alien to traditional Far Eastern diets and is often not tolerated at all.

As an extension of this, a tendency towards certain illnesses varies with populations around the world. Heart disease was hardly ever a problem in Japan, for instance, until the present generation was introduced to Western foods.

Understanding the elements of your constitution makes it much easier to grasp why certain foods have a greater or lesser effect on you. A phlegmatic constitution, for example, tends to produce a lot of mucus. Phlegmatic people may eat a lot of starchy food and dairy products because they like them, and not have any adverse reactions, while someone with a sanguine constitution could be made ill on the same diet. Manipulating our eating habits against our natural constitution is not the right way to go about things, because our constitutional nature digests food in a certain way. Sanguine people are hot and heady, fast-thinking and fast-eating. You can tell them not to eat fast, but you can't say don't think fast. This is their constitution. That's what makes us all different.

Ideally, if we were attuned to our body and were trained by parents and grandparents about healthy cooking and eating, we would know, almost instinctively, exactly what was right for us. But the food industry has created a taste for a lot of wrong things and people no longer generally have this sensitivity. Sometimes adopting a way of eating that is counter to our upbringing or unsuited to the climate or lifestyle can be harmful and result in all sorts of complications, ranging from osteoporosis to a weakened immune system. (In traditional cultures you still see a natural balance and moderation in diet and, as a result, few problems of obesity, heart disease, diabetes, arthritis, irritable bowel syndrome and so on that you see in more 'sophisticated' cultures. Their problems stem more generally from infectious diseases and poor hygiene.)

When it comes to temperament, we are all evolving and changing. Some changes come about with age (teenagers, in particular, are in a constant state of flux) or by a long-term alteration in circumstances. These can be considered permanent shifts and our diet should be modified to cope with them. Other changes are short-term, brought on by anything from emotional stress to jet lag, and here the answer is to cut back or take out those foods that the normal temperament can cope with but the temporarily altered temperament can't. A phlegmatic going through a choleric phase, for instance, may run into problems by eating excess fat and other unsuitable foods, and a shift in diet can counter the stresses and bring about a return to phlegmatism.

the sanguine type

Sanguine people can digest food easily and therefore have a larger range of tolerance. They can consume alcohol in moderation and not be unwell, and do not have to worry about weight problems. However, they need to be aware of sticking within reasonable limits and not abusing their systems because they feel they can eat or drink anything without a problem.

the choleric type

Cholerics have frequent digestive problems; they are the bilious type. They like to drink very cold water because it gives them temporary relief from the heat of the digestive 'fire' within their body. If they eat meat, they should aid its digestion by accompanying it with a lot of raw salad (rocket, lettuce, cucumber, radish or raw onions). The enzymes from these raw foods help to break up meat fibres.

Acidic, fatty and oily foods, and also very sweet, syrupy foods can remain in their stomach for a long time. They tend to burp, have heartburn and can have bad breath from putrefaction. To cope with this tendency, they should eat small amounts of food, chew well, and do some physical movements after eating, particularly after dinner. In short, cholerics are the ones who have to be most cautious about their diet.

the phlegmatic type

The digestion of phlegmatic people is generally good, although very slow. They have sluggish metabolisms and therefore put on weight easily. They may get cravings for sugar, ice cream, cheese, pasta, bread and citrus fruits because they can digest them quickly. Unfortunately these are the very things that produce phlegm or mucus in the body. They can drink alcohol in moderation without ill-effect, but should restrict themselves to red wine and preferably accompany alcohol with protein dishes. They favour hot beverages because these warm them up. Drinking warm water half-an-hour or so after meals is beneficial. Phlegmatics should eat fish, eggs and salads and less fat, and do regular exercise to speed up their digestion and metabolic processes.

the melancholic type

These people have a poor appetite and they can't digest anything heavy – food simply remains in the stomach for a long time. They eat small amounts at a time and like to stick to the same familiar, unchanging foods. Anything that can stimulate their appetite and digestion is welcome: mildly spicy food; an appealing variety of flavours and colours; a small glass of red wine or a tablespoonful of brandy in water half-an-hour before dinner. Jal-Jeera is an Indian mixture of herbs, including cumin, black salt and tamarind that makes a spicy drink which causes the mouth to water and so stimulates the appetite; half a teaspoon of Jal-Jeera powder in a glass of water can help to kick-start the appetite and digestion.

Melancholics have a tendency to avoid protein and become vegetarians, but eating protein is helpful to them.

weight problems

Weight, usually too much of it, is a constant worry to many people – I refer throughout this book about 'diet', meaning 'what we eat', but whenever I talk of diet to a patient, he or she immediately thinks about weight loss. Our diet should be aimed at eating to stay healthy, to prevent and cure illness, not with the sole aim of becoming thinner.

I have seen mothers force-feed their thin children, despite the child's appetite, digestion, elimination and general health being good, because they feel their offspring do not conform to a non-existent norm. People who are by nature fat, fair and flabby (known in an offhand way as FFF), should not spend their whole lives trying to

chapter 14
your health MOT

To focus on what your body requires to be really healthy means you need to stop from time to time for a little self-analysis. You should do this regularly, because your health is such an important aspect of your life: it determines your well-being, your thought processes, your energy levels, your work and your family life. Noticing early signs that you are below par in one area or another and making adjustments to deal with it will keep at bay many chronic problems. To take the analogy of a car, exercising or going on holiday equates with routine servicing, but in addition we need a periodical checkover. I call this My Own Testing, or MOT.

You may already have an annual medical check-up. This will monitor your blood pressure, blood count and cholesterol level, and may include an electrocardiogram (ECG) and some time on a treadmill. Such tests will show up infections and give an indication of fitness, but they tell you little or nothing about your state of health. Employers pay well to find out whether key employees can play their part in running the business; similarly, insurance companies, who will have to pay out if you fall sick, set great store by these annual medicals. In fact, however, they tell you surprisingly little about how capable you are of warding off illness and how well you are able to withstand a job's stresses – just the answers you would think they would need.

So, give yourself the following MOT. The answers will give you enough information to ascertain whether you are very healthy, healthy, borderline, unhealthy or very unhealthy. Let me stress, however, that the purpose of these checks is to determine your state of health, not whether you have any specific ailments. Most people, while not suffering from a particular illness, are not experiencing the vitality and energy of vibrant good health either. Find out where you stand, and how you could improve your level of health and wellbeing.

weight
You need to know three things about your weight:
• Your optimum weight.
• Your normal weight.
• Whether your weight has changed recently, or regularly fluctuates.

Optimum weight A quick rule of thumb to gauge your optimum weight in kilograms is to subtract 100 from your height in centimetres. So a height of 160 cm – 100 = 60 kg.

However, it is an over-simplification to dictate that everyone of 160 cm should weigh 60 kg. This does not take gender, build or musculature into consideration. A better starting point is the World Health Organisation guideline of Body Mass Index (BMI), which allows a range of acceptable weights. But these are still only guidelines – a muscular person could be healthily above average (muscle weighs more than fat), while osteoporosis may give a falsely underweight reading because of light bones.

The death rate from heart disease shows that life expectancy shortens as the BMI rises above 23, so if risks are evident over this figure, then 23 rather than 25 ought to be the upper limit of normal; it has been suggested that the cut-off point of 25 is politically motivated. Interestingly, in Asia it has

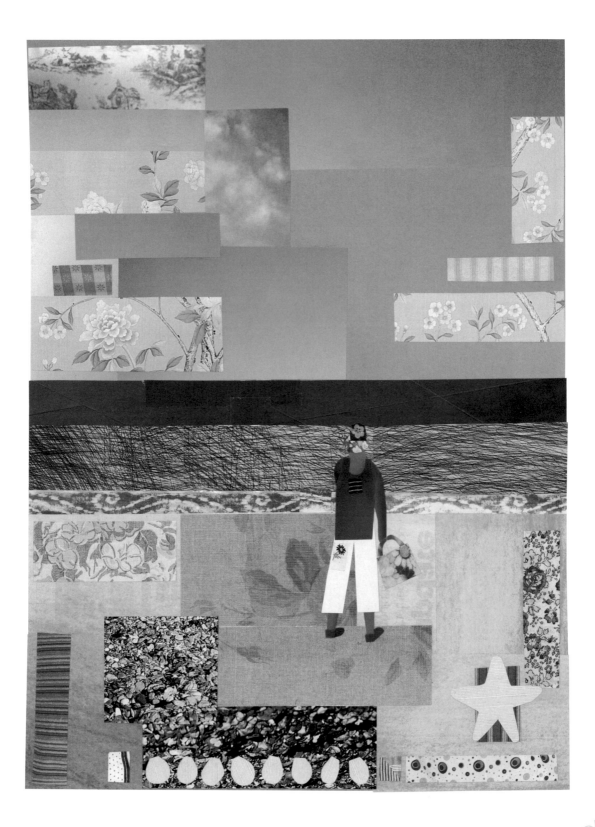

how to calculate your (BMI)

Divide your weight in kilos by the square of your height in metres. Here are a couple of examples:

$57 \text{ kg} \div 1.6 \text{ m}^2 = 57 \div 2.56 = \textbf{22.2}$

$100 \text{ kg} \div 1.85 \text{ m}^2 = 100 \div 3.42 = \textbf{29.2}$

The answers in bold are the BMI (Body Mass Index), which can then be checked against the following ranges:

Underweight	**below 18.5**
Normal	**18.5–24.9**
Overweight	**25.0–29.9**
Obese	**over 30**

You can do these calculations in imperial measures, but the formula is slightly more fiddly: weight in pounds x 704 ÷ (height in inches)[2]

been found that disorders associated with overweight, such as high blood pressure and adult-onset diabetes, occur on average at a lower BMI, and regional obesity guidelines have had to be issued.

Normal weight and weight fluctuations If you weigh yourself regularly you will already know your usual weight. If there is a significant difference between your normal weight and what it should be, you need to do something about it.
Ask yourself the following questions:
• Do you get breathless walking up a flight of stairs?
• When exercising, does your weight cause backstrain?
• Do you often feel lethargic or sluggish, especially in the morning?
• Has your weight increased by 10 per cent or more in the last year?
• (If you have not weighed yourself regularly) Is your clothing tighter than it was, especially round the waist?
• Feel your groin, just above the pubic bone. Is the area very sore?

If the answer to any of these is Yes, then you are probably overweight. Read pages 123–5 for further guidance.

Another useful factor to check is your waist measurement. Measurements above 85 cm for a woman or 100 cm for a man, or a waist that keeps expanding, indicate a need to lose weight. Measurements are a little subjective here, as you will need to assess whether to allow for anything like temporary abdominal bloating, weak muscles or herniation.

As important as the actual weight is a noticeable variation in weight. Such fluctuations could indicate unsuitable on–off dieting (see page 125) or a metabolic imbalance (see Chapter 16).

pulse, breathing and blood pressure

These are three other body measurements you can determine yourself. They should all be taken while you are at rest, so sit down quietly for a few minutes before you begin.

pulse rate

Put three fingers (not your thumb) of one hand on the wrist of the other hand, just below the base of the thumb. Ensure you can clearly feel your pulse beating. Use a watch that counts seconds to check the number of beats per minute.
below 60 Slow but not of concern (sports enthusiasts will generally have a slower pulse rate as their bodies have adapted to regulating their pulse when exercising hard).
60–75 Normal.
over 80 Cause for concern.
irregular Get yourself checked by a professional.

breathing rate

Put your hand on top of your abdomen, school yourself to breathe regularly (it's easy to pant or hold your breath when you make yourself conscious of your breathing) and time your in-breaths for a minute. The rate should be around 16 per minute. If it is much more than this you are hyperventilating – this could be a nervous reaction (test yourself several times), or it could mean that excess abdominal gas is lifting the diaphragm and not leaving you enough room to breathe deeply. It may also indicate a heart or lung problem.

blood pressure

Your blood pressure is gauged by two readings, systolic (the higher figure) and diastolic (the lower), taken as the heart contracts and relaxes in its work of pumping blood around the body. There are a number of meters on the market for reading your own blood pressure, but some are more accurate than others, and unless you have been trained it is easy to get a wrong reading – which may send up your blood pressure unnecessarily! It is becoming ever easier to get your blood pressure checked by a trained professional without making a doctor's appointment: you can go to drop-in surgeries, well woman/well man clinics and facilities at pharmacies.

When you are relaxed the levels should be between 120/70 and 135/85 if you are under 40, but blood pressure tends to rise with age and higher readings can be considered normal.

age range	highest 'normal' pressure readings
20–40	135/85
40–60	140/85
60–80	150/90

A diastolic pressure of below 60 or above 90 is outside the normal range at any age.

If your blood pressure falls outside the range of normal for your age, consult a health professional.

energy

Fatigue is one of the most injurious conditions to health. Lack of energy is like a power failure in the body. The liver will not function well, your absorption, circulation and kidney function will be poor, your muscles will be atonic and you will be prone to depression. It is one thing to be aware that your energy is limited and to conserve it accordingly, to accept some tiredness at night,

but regular exhaustion is bad. Check your energy by considering the following questions:

On waking, do you:
• Leap out of bed with vitality?
• Ease out like a snail from his shell?

By an hour after lunch are you:
• Still full of beans?
• Ready to call it a day?

By the end of the day, do you:
• Feel the day has really taken its toll?
• Still feel game for more?

We get energy from food and we regain our energy from sleep. If you normally feel lethargic, then take a closer look at what you are eating and reread the book so far, in particular the parts that relate to your lifestyle. In addition, consider your pattern and quality of sleep.

sleep

Years ago we thought we needed eight hours' sleep a night. For some reason this has generally gone down to six. What is important is the quality of sleep. This may depend on your lifestyle. Ask yourself about how you sleep:
• How many hours a night do you usually sleep?
• Has your sleep pattern changed recently?
• Do you wake up refreshed or tired?

Continuous sleep is not essential and it can be averaged. Three really good nights' sleep in a week will compensate for other nights that are restless or wakeful to some extent, but less than four hours is not good. Dark circles under your eyes, when you are not suffering from a chronic debilitating illness or anaemia, indicate lack of restful sleep.

Some causes of broken sleep or sleeplessness are easier to rectify than others, and most are outside the scope of this book, but digestion can also be a factor (see pages 205–7).

digestion

Do you have a bowel movement every day?
It is not necessary to evacuate at the same time every day, but your bowels should move every

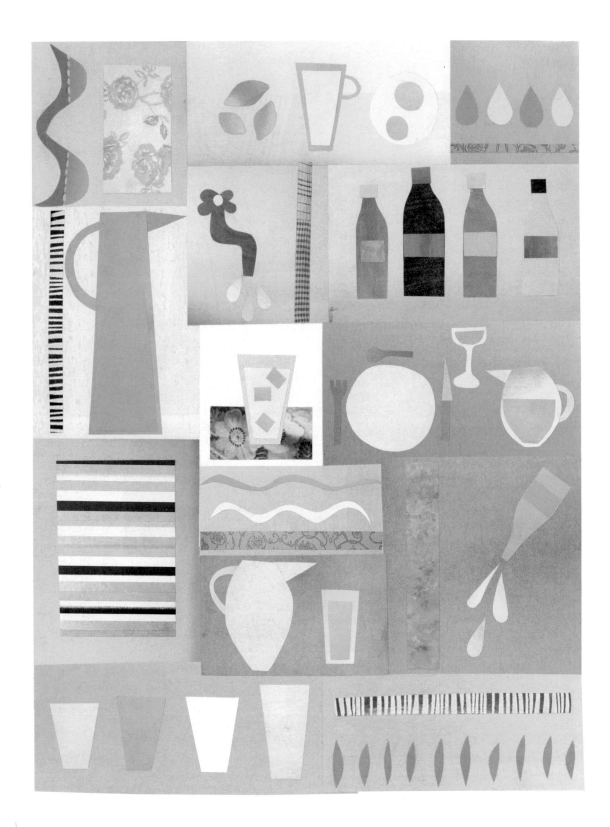

24 hours or so. Chronic constipation can be an indication of several health problems, and also create them (see pages 140–44).

Do you experience excessive flatulence or burping? Do you feel bloated after meals?
Eating too fast, producing too much acid, irregular meals, fizzy drinks and stress can all create excessive wind – by which I mean enough for you or another to remark on. (See chapters 3, 4 and 15 in particular.)

Is your urine almost colourless or dark? Does it smell strongly?
Urine should be clear or pale yellow with no strong smell. If it is very yellow you are not drinking enough water. Certain foods such as beetroot or asparagus can taint your urine but this should only be a temporary quirk that quickly passes. Strong-smelling urine may indicate an excess of vitamins (particularly B) or protein.

Is there a burning sensation when you pass urine?
You may not be drinking enough water or your diet may be too highly spiced or acidic (see pages 40–41). Alternatively, you may be suffering from thrush (see page 191) or a urinary tract infection (see page 155).

Problems with urinating should be checked out with a professional as they may be indicative of a range of disorders, from an enlarged prostate to kidney malfunction.

How does your breath smell?
The vapours from the stomach come up continuously into the mouth. Blow from deep down into your palm and sniff.

A rotten egg or ammonia smell? A sign of putrefaction in your gums or your stomach. It could be caused by excess protein or failing to digest properly, or it may be emanating from pus from gumboils, gingivitis or pyorrhoea. Oral hygiene is very important.

A sweet or acetone (nail varnish) smell? This indicates you are eating too much carbohydrate – it is caused by excess yeast and fermenting alcohol in the stomach.

These are the two main smells, though a physician can detect a lot more. If your breath doesn't smell fresh, see pages 148 and 184.

what your tongue says about your health
The tongue is a reflection of the body. By examining it you can diagnose various health conditions, including anaemia, dehydration, presence of gut yeast or fungus, constipation, acidity, liver malfunction and stomach ulcers. Sit in front of a mirror and study your tongue.

Is the back of your tongue furry?
This indicates excessive acid or that you are not evacuating toxins well enough (constipation may be the reason). Acid also produces a smooth narrow red band round the edge of the tongue. (Also see page 27.)

Are there any small ulcerations or cracks, particularly in the central part?
These may mean your liver is sluggish or you have excess yeast in the gut (see pages 44–5 and 151).

Is the tip reddish?
You are eating too many carbohydrates (see page 13).

Does it look slightly shrivelled?
You are not drinking enough water (see pages 24–5).

Does your tongue have impressions of the teeth either side?
Gastric upsets can expand your tongue so much that it presses against the sides of the teeth.

what your eyes say about your health
Bright-eyed? Bleary-eyed? Red-eyed? We all know that our eyes reflect how we are feeling. A whole science – iridology – has grown up devoted to

diagnosing health problems via tell-tale signs in the iris, but you don't need to be an expert to deduce a few things from your sclera (the whites of your eyes).

• Tenseness will slightly shrivel the small blood vessels in the sclera.

• A long period of stress (which may include sleeplessness) or an overload of toxins in the system will cause these blood vessels to burst. If this has happened recently the eyes will appear bloodshot.

• If the situation continues the iron in the blood will turn brownish (just like a scab on your skin does). Definitely time you took remedial action.

what your skin says about your health

The state of your skin is a good guide to your digestive health.

An overall **dry skin** – not just rough patches due to exposure or flaky areas (see below) – may be caused by washing away natural oils or a dietary deficiency. Ask yourself:

• Am I bathing in over-hot water, thereby removing too much of the skin's natural lubrication?

• Is the soap or skin cleanser I'm using too harsh?

• How much oil am I consuming? If sufficient, is my liver digesting properly or not? Oil needs to be balanced, not too much or too little – a maximum of 4 tbsp of olive oil in cooking per day is a useful rule of thumb.

• If none of these seem to provide the answer, it could be a vitamin deficiency. Put mustard oil under your toenails and in your umbilicus (navel). Goodness knows how it distributes, but it works.

When the body eliminates fat-soluble toxins via the sebaceous glands, excess sebum can leave skin **greasy** or **oily**. Over-excited sebaceous glands can upset the uppermost layer of skin, causing it to become **itchy** or **scaly**. This also leads to 'barber's itch' in the beard area on men. The skin may then seem dry, but the flakes are, in fact, saturated with oil. Blackheads and acne are also a result of overactive sebaceous glands (see Chapter 20).

The skin around the nose is dense with sebaceous glands, and a chronically **red nose**, even when it's warm, indicates you have too much yeast in your system or you have been drinking too much.

Itchiness can be due to excessive garlic or salt.

Soreness at the corners of the mouth can be caused by vitamin deficiency, particularly of vitamins A and B.

Bluish white spots on arms and legs and body (in considerable quantity, not one or two) indicates a high acid content in the stomach and hyperactivity of the pancreas. People who eat too much and too fast get these marks.

Brownish patches on the cheeks can indicate chronic anaemia or liver malfunction.

Grey patches on the face (prominent in growing children) indicates calcium deficiency.

what your hair and nails reveal

Your hair, like your skin, is a reflection of inner health. Washing will clean it and a conditioner will add a superficial gloss, but because hair is already dead nothing you apply to it will make it intrinsically healthier; this can only be done internally. When we are ill, or chronically below par or stressed, this shows in dull, out-of-condition hair.

A sudden increase in **hair loss** could indicate a nutritional deficiency, low blood pressure or other restriction that means the scalp is not getting as much oxygenated blood as it should, a hormonal imbalance or stress. A **fungal infection**, such as alopecia, can also account for hair falling out in unusual amounts (see page 184).

Dandruff or flaking scalp is caused by sebaceous glands working overtime (see page 182). A **dry, itchy scalp** that is not caused by dandruff may be due to zinc deficiency.

Diagnostic hair testing is a good indicator of any past deficiency of minerals but doesn't necessarily reflect your current state of health.

Nails take about four months to grow from the base to the top, so in them you can see a history of your recent state of health. A horizontal ridge or indentation, for instance, shows an interruption in the nail's growth that records a disruption in your health, and where it occurs indicates how long ago it was (so halfway up your nail would be about two months ago). Study your nails periodically to see what they tell you:

• A series of horizontal bands: a long period or continuing ill-health or poor nutrition.
• White patches: a mineral deficiency (though not necessarily, as is commonly believed, of calcium; zinc is more likely).
• Vertical streaks: a sign of ongoing chronic disease.

Nails can also be prey to fungal infections (see pages 184–5).

your drinking habits
fluids
How much water do you drink a day?
Water is important for keeping our various bodily systems functioning well and for helping flush out toxins. Aim to drink around 2 litres a day (see pages 24–5 and illustration on page 130).

alcohol
The stresses that excess alcohol puts on your body, and the damage it does are covered in Chapter 4. Tolerance to alcohol is a very individual thing. This is not the same as a heavy drinker requiring a greater amount of alcohol before feeling the effects. It is how efficient your body is at processing alcohol and eliminating it from the blood. Try this test:

1 Choose a time when you have an empty stomach and can sit quietly somewhere for at least half-an-hour.
2 Pour yourself a glass of wine (175 ml). Before drinking any wine, make a note of the time and your pulse rate.
3 Sip the wine slowly over the next half hour. You can read a book or listen to music during this time, but don't do anything that might raise your pulse rate, such as watching an exciting TV programme or getting involved in a stimulating conversation.
4 Every 10 minutes measure your pulse (see page 128) and write it down.

If, after 10 minutes, it is 10 per cent above the first measurement, you are absorbing the alcohol. Your pulse should peak at the 10- or 20-minute check at not more than 40 per cent of the base level and then stabilise at that rate.

If the peak rises above 40 per cent of the base then you are reacting to the alcohol. It will remain like this for 30–40 minutes. This shows you are sensitive to it. If during this period you get any symptoms like headaches or dizziness then you are overreacting. The chances are either that you are addictive, that you have some problem with your liver that is making its processing slow, or that excessive yeast in your gut is producing its own alcohol.

If your pulse stabilised well, try the experiment again, but double the amount of wine to 1½ or 2 glasses over a half-hour period.

This raising and relaxing of the pulse is similar to what happens during vigorous exercise – someone who is very fit will be able to sustain greater effort before reaching a pulse rate of, say, 100, and it will more quickly fall back to the normal resting rate.

By graduated steps you can measure how well your body processes alcohol; everyone is different. You will also get a different reaction if you have recently eaten.

your lifestyle
The above questions and observations relate principally to diet and nutrition. Every part of your life is interrelated, however, so look at the whole picture by similarly examining:

• Exercise: how regularly do you exercise? Is it giving you a good workout without straining you?
• Stress: how much do you have? How well do you cope with decision-making, conflict or unexpected change?
• Relaxation: are you a workaholic? When did you last have a holiday, a massage or learn or do something quite new and different?

Give yourself a complete MOT every six weeks or so. This way you will get to know the workings of your body and take conscious note of how a healthier diet has reverberations all through your life.

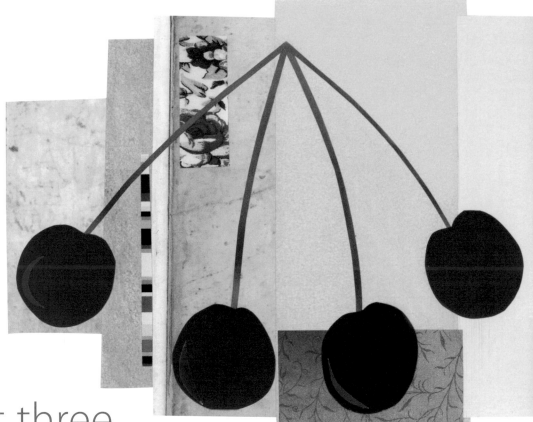

part three
when things
go wrong

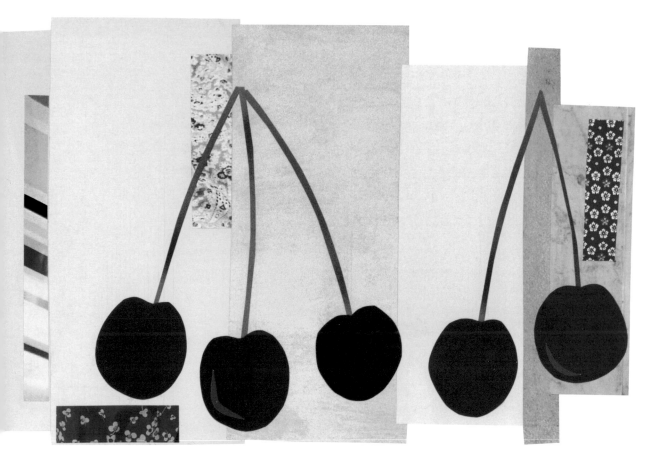

When I hear Ashkanazi play Chopin or Ustad Sultan Khan play a raga or watch an Olympic gymnast perform I wonder how we doctors can be so insensitive as to treat anything as beautiful as the human miracle with a packet of pills or a knife. The human body requires tender loving care, and who is better motivated to administer that to your own body than you?

integrated health

Up to now we have focused on the most important part of medicine, the maintenance and optimising of health through nutrition. If this were a hundred per cent successful there would be no need for treatment of disease and hospitals would be empty. This is not a perfect world, however, and things do go wrong, so this third part of the book is about the management of sickness. This is when TLC is really needed.

Just as health results from the careful balancing of the body's systems, so diseases are the result of the lowering of the sanogenetic defences, allowing pathogens such as bacteria or viruses to attack one or more of those systems, throwing them out of balance. How do we restore the balance and effect a cure? Do we boost the defences, or do we attack the pathogens? Do we treat the diseased, or the disease?

Immediately we come to the parting of the ways between conventional and integrated medicine. Conventional medicine treats the disease, often ignoring the individuality of the patient, and even the cause, in the blind rush to recreate normality. Integrated medicine treats the patient as an individual and a cooperative partner to restore health and therefore fight off the disease. You have to be involved. You may sometimes need that packet of pills but eighty per cent of the healing will still come from you, mostly through nutritional care, with exercise and therapeutic massage as well.

Conventional medicine is called allopathic, from *allo* (other), *patho* (agent of disease). In other words, conventional medicine introduces other pathogens, usually toxins (in the case of drugs or chemotherapy) to counter the first pathogen (the disease). Integrated medicine adjusts the lifestyle of the patient (the diseased) to restore the defensive network and the balance of the systems to their healthy state. Conventional medicine therefore requires least effort from the patient, who simply remains passive. Some conventional treatments even suppress the body's own efforts at healing, such as the secretion of natural steroids. Integrated medicine is harder on the patient because it demands full cooperation and effort to build up those defences, but with a far higher ultimate reward – good health.

Diagnosis

I firmly believe that one should not treat without a definite diagnosis in mind. If making such a diagnosis is difficult on a patient's first visit, I take my time and ponder over it until the next visit. In the meantime I recommend Regimen Therapy (see chapter 7), which is just sensible dietary and exercise advice, to see if there are more clues to the actual cause of the complaint.

Most illnesses are multifactorial. Influenza, for example, involves weakening of the defences, the presence of a virulent agent, the weakening of the lining of the nasal tract, headache, muscle ache and fatigue, all apparently unconnected. Conventional medicine has no convenient answer to a multifactorial illness, since drugs are designed to hit a particular pathogen, so numerous symptoms require as many drugs to hit each. They say if you don't treat flu you will heal in a week but if you do treat it you'll heal in seven days. The fact is most diseases heal on their own if the right conditions are set up. Drugs only help the body in about 20 per cent of cases. Integrated medicine employs the body's own healing agents which tackle all the factors. In many cases general treatment in the form of Regimen Therapy, perhaps supplemented with a tonic, is the only treatment needed, and it is one that everyone can apply the moment they feel ill with absolutely no risk and a good chance of success.

Often, however, it is the single symptoms that cause concern. These are warning signs that your body has reached a threshold or that it is fighting off an 'invader'.

Pain is perhaps the most obvious. Everybody experiences pain from time to time, and minor pains – stiffness from exercise, jaw ache from chewing nuts, occasional cramp – we live with without concern. If, however, pain is continuous or regular or it wakes you up at night, or worries you because you don't know the cause, you need to seek advice.

Another common symptom that something is wrong is fever. As well as sweating and feeling your temperature is out of control, your heart rate and anxiety level go up, you feel sluggish, your muscles and whole body ache. The symptoms restrict you and make you slow down, which is one of the things your body needs in order to garner strength to fight the cause of the fever. A viral fever may be accompanied by a runny nose, headache, muscular fatigue, cold congestion or slight irritation in the throat. A doctor should be consulted for a high fever that brings on delirium or for a recurrent fever at a particular time. In children and the elderly a fever lasting longer than 24 hours requires medical help, and for other adults 3–4 days is the limit. Within these limits rest, warmth and a mild diet are sufficient. Don't try to reduce the temperature with drugs, unless it is very high (when the doctor should be involved anyway). Raising its temperature is the body's way of limiting pathogens, which cannot survive at the higher temperature. When the fever goes down it shows the body's sanogenetic forces have overcome the invading pathogen, but the task of healing is not complete. Recuperation afterwards is most important.

I have made references to seeking medical help.

As a simple rule of thumb: if the condition is acute (sudden and severe) go to a conventional doctor; if it is chronic (persistent) go to an integrated or complementary physician. In areas without such a clinic, however, the responsibility of which treatment to seek falls on you. This is perhaps the major failing of the health service – that such a critical decision should be left to the patient. It results too often in an automatic fallback on conventional medicine, and is probably the major cause of overrun in the health budget.

Integrated medicine

In an integrated clinic you will first meet a skilled diagnostician and generalist ('a gatekeeper') who will direct you to the most appropriate physician. Just as most forms of ill-health are multifactorial, integrated medicine is multi-disciplinary and will bring in whatever form of therapy is best suited to the illness and the patient.

At the Integrated Medical Centre we use conventional medicine as and when required. I would estimate that about a third of our therapy is conventional: antibiotics, diuretics, painkillers, anti-histamines, and, occasionally, tranquillisers and vitamins and minerals in injectable form. We use the latter particularly for cancer therapies (because of poor appetite and the need to nourish the body with essentials), chronic fatigue syndrome (because of poor absorption) and during convalescence. In psychiatry we use psychological medicine, neurolinguistic programming (NLP), hypnosis, different types of psychological treatment and conventional medicines depending on the acuteness of the disease.

The prime recommendation, though, before any further treatment, is Regimen Therapy (see chapter 7). Much of the lifestyle programme in integrated health is concerned with diet, because so much of the activities of the body depend on the efficiency of digestion. Too many people treat their stomachs as the municipal garbage dump and suffer more than they realise, which is why adopting a healthy diet so often works wonders.

Once the patient feels good all the body's self-regulatory processes are geared up to restore the balance in the body and repair the damage done by a disease. In this situation the body is well prepared for self-healing. The power of Regimen Therapy is such that often I am reluctant to use any other treatment, however non-invasive or safe. When required, however, integrated medicine draws on many different forms of therapy. These include:

Naturopathy

A mixture of diet, massage, water hydrotherapy and some juices, without the use of herbal, homeopathic or any chemical medicines. This is often the best course for chronic ailments such as eczema, asthma, gastritis, psoriasis, arthritis and liver disorders.

Acupuncture

Stimulating precise points on the body has long been recognised as an effective method of reducing pain and re-establishing the body's equilibrium. Inserting fine needles into the skin is, contrary to what you might expect, painless. Among other things it releases endorphins, which are the body's own form of morphine and are excellent painkillers. It is used in hospitals for terminal cancer pain, and I use it for back pain, arthritic pains and migraine.

Apart from its painkilling properties it is used for stimulating energy, can help regulate the systems of the body (particularly the autonomous nervous system), inflammation, mild hypertension (high blood pressure), panic attacks, insomnia, anxiety, itchiness, tinnitus, deafness, loss of smell, tingling and numbness in the fingers due to some neurological problem, post-operative conditions, loss of sensation, nerve-related conditions such as Bell's palsy, paralysis, stroke etc., stomach ulcers and double vision. Moxibustion is used in some instances to increase the effectiveness of the needles by heat, and acupressure stimulates the same trigger points by fingertip pressure rather than needles.

Homeopathy

Homeopathy is glibly described as 'treating like with like' – which is true, but not very helpful in understanding how it works. It uses natural remedies in minute doses and involves much careful diagnosis of the patient's type as well as the symptoms. A good homeopathic physician holds a bunch of keys and knows exactly which key to fit into the lock of an ailment to open it. Homeopathy is at its best with allergies, such as asthma, eczema and hay fever. We use it for problems of the mind (depression, anxiety and insomnia), warts, corns, benign growths, tonsilitis, acute flu (it works on the energy system of the body and builds up immunity), acidity, irritable bowel syndrome (if not connected with any food intolerances), rheumatoid arthritis and some auto-immune problems. In general it is most effective where the constitution or whole body needs to be built up. A feature of almost all healing to a greater or lesser extent is the 'healing crisis' (see page 60), but it is perhaps more pronounced in homeopathy.

Herbal remedies

Ayurvedic, Chinese and Unani herbal medicines are outstanding in treatment of liver disorders such as hepatitis (particularly hepatitis C, for which conventional medicine is sadly weak). We also use them for chronic sinus problems, eczema (again, no conventional equivalent) and irritable bowel syndrome. The only remedy available for constipation is selenium husk, or senna, which is also used in conventional medicine.

We also use herbs for impotence, infertility, hypertension, toning up the heart and circulatory system, and as a general tonic. There is not much money in herbal tonics so nowadays conventional medicine has turned to vitamin B complexes and other supplements, which bring a much better return to the drug companies, but herbal tonics are just as effective. We use herbal remedies for urinary infections and kidney stones (though not gall stones). Ayurvedic oils with anti-inflammatory properties are used in oil baths to help arthritis, and chronic sciatica and backache. Oil massage of the head has a soothing effect on the brain, a powerful psychotherapeutic effect and induces sleep.

Specific therapeutic yoga

Used for clearing sinuses and bowels, which are affected by a number of ailments. Yoga as an enormously effective 'medicine' and route to good health is covered fully in my book *Therapeutic Yoga* (see page 220).

Colonic hydrotherapy

This is useful to aid healing and eliminate toxins to cure conditions such as constipation and accumulation of gas and toxins.

Osteopathy and Chiropractic

We use these forms of manipulative therapy for any subluxation (dislocation) of joints. Although exercise and massage can normally clear such problems, patients usually want speedy relief, especially if they can't walk, move or function in some way. Manipulation is often miraculous in its speed. Cranial osteopathy, which we also use, is slow and very gentle, but improves circulation of blood and cerebral fluid to the brain, on the principle that if the brain functions better the rest of the body functions better too.

Healing by touch

There is a significant link between a physician and patient when contact is made. All doctors who touch their patients practise healing to some degree. When I have completed a period of, say, neck massage, I feel strangely drained of energy. Though I recover quite quickly it is a very noticeable effect. There is no question in my experience that healing through the hands is an effective therapy. We use it very often in relief of chronic or unexplained pains, double vision, stroke victims and, to some degree, with multiple sclerosis. I would say that it brings about necessary change in the tissues to kick-start the healing

process, not unlike jump-starting a car so that you can charge up the battery by running the engine.

We also use, when appropriate, chiropody, podiatry and, to clear arteries of a build up of plaque, chelation therapy.

Selecting the form of treatment for a particular ailment, however, is is not always as straightforward as this may make it sound. For example, eczema can be treated by homeopathy as well as Ayurvedic herbal medicines. I would normally choose the latter as it is quicker to treat it with a selection of herbs than depend on the trial method of selection of the constitutional homoeopathic remedy. On the other hand, herbal medicines may not taste pleasant or may be fiddly to prepare and may occasionally give undesirable side-effects like loose bowel movements. Homeopathy rarely produces any side-effects.

Over the years I have formed a 'protocol' of treatments for various diseases. Based on my own experience and those of my colleagues at the Integrated Medical Centre, carefully observing the reactions of different types of treatment, these protocols are working modules and can be used as standardised methods of treatments for various ailments. It does not mean that the individual is ignored. The physician's skills are needed in introducing variations in these protocols, and in tailoring treatment to the patient. For example, if someone is scared of needles then acupuncture is not the best form of treatment because it will create emotional problems. Other factors, such as cost, availability of herbs or remedies, experience of the specialist and individual response to the treatment, all need to be taken into account.

This book is about nutrition. Obviously nutrition may be insufficient on its own, and the diets and regimes I recommend may need to be backed up by one of the treatments described above. But nutrition is at the heart of health. Nutrition therapy is not one you will normally be prescribed by a conventional doctor. If you embark on it you are most likely seeking an integrated cure, so the following chapters need to be read with this in mind.

chapter 15
digestive and urinary health

The moment you put something in your mouth there is an impact on your health, positive or negative. The digestive system is the warehouse for the whole body, supplying nutrients to every other system. It is also responsible for the disposal of most of the body's waste products. When something goes wrong with the digestive system, the whole body can be affected. If you have any digestive problems, reread Chapter 2, as understanding how your digestion works is key to understanding what is going wrong.

CONSTIPATION

Just as we eat every day so, in principle, we should evacuate our bowels daily. The odd irregularity is of no consequence, but chronic constipation – when passing stools less than four times a week is the norm – gives rise to all sorts of associated problems: excess flatulence; abdominal cramps; a full, heavy abdomen leading to poor appetite; calcium and magnesium deficiency (absorption from dry or hard stools is difficult); the growth of polyps and tumours; haemorrhoids or piles from straining to produce a bowel movement; anal fissures from dry bowels; headaches; and sinus problems. This last occurs because toxins are not being eliminated in the usual way, so the body channels them instead into the sinuses to be expelled, resulting in a build-up of mucus in the sinus cavity.

Constipation can be caused directly by certain foods or a lack of them, but chronic constipation often has its source in a habitual problem that may even date back to childhood. Worry and stress, being rushed in the morning, perhaps due to queues for the family toilet or leaving too little time to get ready for work, and sitting in the toilet for too long because of distractions such as reading, can all lead to sluggish bowel movements.

Sometimes constipation can be relieved suddenly with a bout of diarrhoea – which may be brought about by the amount of water, fibre, spices or laxatives consumed. This may also indicate irritable bowel syndrome (see pages 150–54). A regular pattern of constipation alternating with diarrhoea may be caused by diverticular disease (see page 149).

Dietary guidance

Your diet plays an important role in the treatment of constipation. Although eating roughage for bowel movements works for most people, the interesting thing is that different foodstuffs help to ease the bowels in different people. Many find the following help:
• Chillies or spicy food. Spices facilitate bowel movements, and chillies are known to irritate the lining of the gut and so more saliva and mucus are produced, helping to soften stools. In fact, they cause diarrhoea in many people. Chillies also stimulate appetites by increasing gastric secretion.
• Milk. This is a mild laxative, especially the full-cream variety, but in the many people intolerant to lactose (milk sugar) it brings on diarrhoea, which in a constipated gut means a good bowel movement.

• Yoghurt. This works in the same way as milk, and the bacteria in live yoghurt help ease digestion.
• Satsumas, clementines and oranges. Eating these fruits (with pith and pips, not just the juice) helps to ease bowel movements in some people. The seeds and fibres have anti-binding properties that help to keep stools soft.

Meal suggestions to ease constipation

Breakfast
• High-fibre cereals with warm cow's milk (or soya milk if lactose-intolerant).
• Prunes, raisins, dried apricots and figs soaked overnight. Chop them and a banana and mix into plain live yoghurt.
Add honey or molasses to either of the above.

Main meals
Overleaf you'll find some recipes for dishes that can help to relieve constipation.

Helpful nutritional supplements

• 1 cup of fresh aloe vera juice twice a day is a good tonic for constipation.

food solutions for constipation
The following foods have natural laxative properties, so include a selection in your diet if you need to loosen your bowels.

prunes	okra
kiwi fruit	spinach
rhubarb	high-fibre cereals
bananas	linseed
figs	sesame seeds
grapes	molasses
courgettes	porridge
beetroot	pepper
yams	pumpkins
chickpeas	cabbage
cucumber	

Other beneficial treatments

• Yoga poses such as the Child's Pose (see my book *Therapeutic Yoga*, page 220), will help ease the bowels.

piles (haemorrhoids)
Straining to evacuate your bowels damages the sensitive anal veins, allowing blood to accumulate in them – piles are varicose veins in the anus. They begin inside the anus, where they may bleed and itch, but once they protrude out into the air they will dry up and are more likely to bleed, causing greater discomfort and, during a bowel movement, extreme pain.

As it is straining that induces piles, the answer is to cure the constipation that necessitates it (see above). To relieve the pain until the piles shrink back to normal, use moist toilet tissue, and try to keep the piles from drying out by pushing them back into the anus. Contract the anus about 20 times two or three times a day, to improve circulation in that area, and dull the pain with ice cubes.

recipes to relieve constipation

spicy spinach and lentils

1 cup lentils, soaked and rinsed
  (see page 50)
250–400 g fresh spinach,
  chopped (or frozen equivalent)
thumb-sized piece root ginger
3 tbsp olive oil
2 cloves garlic, chopped
½ tsp mustard seeds
½ tsp cumin seeds
½ tsp fenugreek seeds
1 medium onion, chopped
2 tomatoes, chopped
½–1 tsp salt
½ tsp mild chilli powder
  or black pepper

1 Bring the lentils to the boil in 4 cups of water. Add the spinach and ginger and continue to boil for 20 minutes until you have a porridge-like mixture.

2 Heat the oil in a frying pan and fry the garlic, mustard, cumin and fenugreek on a high heat for 10 seconds. Add the onion and tomatoes and cook gently until the onions are light brown. Add 2 cups of the lentil and spinach mixture to the pan and stir for 30 seconds to incorporate the spice mix.

3 Return this to the main lentil pot and cook for a further 2 minutes, stirring the spices through the mixture. Add salt and chilli or pepper to taste.

spicy mixed vegetables

1 medium aubergine
2 tomatoes
250 g red pumpkin
250 g fresh spinach
1 large sweet pepper
1 medium onion
2 cloves garlic
4 tsp olive oil
½ tsp black cumin seeds
½ tsp aniseed
pinch of asafoetida (available
  in Indian grocery shops or
  by mail order)
¼ tsp ground black pepper
½–1 tsp salt

1 Chop all the vegetables separately into even-sized dice. Heat the oil to medium hot in a pan. Add the black cumin, aniseed and asafoetida and fry, stirring, for 10 seconds. Add the onion and garlic and fry until they are light brown. Add the rest of the vegetables, and pepper and salt to taste, and stir together well.

2 Cover and cook over a low heat for about 20–25 minutes until the vegetables are soft. Sprinkle with a little water from time to time to produce steam and keep the mixture moist, and stir to avoid the vegetables sticking to the pan.

herby chicken or fish

100 g coriander leaves
6 cloves garlic
2–4 medium-hot fresh chillies
1 medium onion, quartered
4 tbsp olive oil
250 g chicken breast, diced,
    or fillet of fish cut in finger
    lengths
½–1 tsp salt

1 Blend together the coriander, garlic, chillies and onion with 1 tbsp of water to make a green paste.

2 Heat the oil in a frying pan and fry the paste on a medium heat, stirring often, for 7–10 minutes. Add the chicken or fish, stir to mix into the spice mixture, add salt to taste and simmer gently until just cooked. The chicken will take 10–15 minutes, and the fish 5–7 minutes.

3 Leave to cool, then reheat thoroughly before serving; this will ensure the flavour penetrates the chicken or fish.

spiced okra

250 g okra
3 tbsp olive oil
¼ tsp cumin seeds
¼ tsp mustard seeds
1 medium onion, chopped
2 cloves garlic
½ tsp salt
¼ tsp hot chilli powder or
    ground black pepper
2 tomatoes

1 Chop the okra into 1-cm lengths at the last minute to prevent the viscous juice it exudes from becoming too sticky.

2 Heat the oil in a frying pan and fry the cumin and mustard seeds over a medium heat for 10 seconds. Add the onion, okra (and its juice) and garlic and fry until brown, stirring regularly.

3 Add salt to taste and the chilli or black pepper, stir and cook for 1 minute then add the tomatoes. Cover and simmer for 3–5 minutes.

soothing infusions to relieve constipation

The following infusions will help to relieve the uncomfortable symptoms of constipation, such as abdominal cramps and excess flatulence.

Ginger tea Chop or slice a thumb-sized piece of root ginger and boil in 2 cups of water for 5 minutes. Add 1 tsp of tea leaves and boil for a further 20 seconds. Stir in a few crystals of salt to stabilise the taste and reduce the pungency of the ginger. You can drink it plain, with a slice of lemon or with honey or warm milk. Add a pinch of black pepper for a more potent effect. Taken at bedtime, especially with the added pepper, this is a very useful bowel tonic for the next morning.

Psyllium milk Mix 2 tbsp of psyllium husks (also known as isaphogol) in 2 cups of warm water and stir quickly. Add 1 tsp of honey or molasses sugar and drink quickly as it becomes thicker by the second. Follow it a couple of minutes later with a glass of water. Take 2–3 hours after dinner or at bedtime. Some traditional physicians recommend psyllium husk with milk. As milk neutralises stomach acid it slows down digestion, so it is especially important to allow 2–3 hours to elapse after a meal. This is also helpful in clearing partially digested food and alcohol from the intestines if you have overeaten or had too much to drink.

Tukmaria Soak 1 tsp of these black seeds in 250 ml or a tumblerful of organic apple or grape juice or plain water for about an hour. The seeds will swell up. Drink on an empty stomach or 2–3 hours after a meal. The taste is bland, but you can add 1 tsp of honey or molasses sugar if you like.

FLATULENCE

Flatulence can be uncomfortable, embarrassing and yet so easily minimalised. Causes include: constipation, fermentation and other chemical reactions in the gut, and putrefaction from the action of bacteria on protein or nitrogenous products in the gut, producing ammoniacal or sulphuric-smelling gas.

No one is immune from occasional flatulence, but regular and excessive build-up of gas in the colon can raise the diaphragm and cause breathlessness, or push the stomach upwards enhancing the formation of hiatus hernia (see page 151). Internal pressures like this can also cause backache.

Dietary guidance

You should avoid the following:
• Coffee.
• Fizzy drinks, including champagne and carbonated water.
• Yeast products.
• Beer (which is both fizzy and yeasty).
• Fibrous stalks of stems of asparagus, broccoli and cauliflower.
• Cereals high in insoluble fibre (roughage) (see pages 13–14).
• Radishes.
• Chickpeas.
• Canned foods.
• Sugars (which feed fermentation in the gut).

Instead, eat:
• Beetroot.
• Papaya.
• Carrots.
• Garlic (chop a clove or two of raw garlic and swallow with water).

Also try the following drinks:
• Peppermint tea.
• Ginger tea (see opposite).
• Carrot juice.
• Fenugreek water (1 tsp of seeds soaked overnight in a glass of warm water).

Helpful nutritional supplements

Two Indian herbs that are particularly effective in reducing flatulence are:
• Kalonji (*Nigella sativa*): Boil 1 tsp of seeds in a glassful of water for 5 minutes. Leave to infuse for another 5 minutes before drinking. Sometimes kalonji seeds are put in Asian and Middle Eastern breads to help counteract the gas-producing effect of the yeast. You can buy kalonji in Indian grocery stores; they are often labelled black cumin (bigger and darker than real cumin). Onion seed is also sometimes called kalonji and this works well too.
• Kadu (*Helleborus niger*): Helps eliminate gut yeast and fungus, which are common sources of flatulence. It is also a mild purgative, so helps the evacuation of gases. Soak two or three twigs in a cup of hot water overnight. Strain and drink on an empty stomach in the morning.

Other beneficial treatments

• Massage the abdomen with sesame oil in a clockwise fashion.
• Adopt the yoga wind-relieving pose (see my book, *Therapeutic Yoga*, page 220).

DIARRHOEA

Sudden diarrhoea accompanied by vomiting or a fever may be caused by food poisoning and should always be checked out by a doctor. However, if you just have very runny stools, give your body a chance to put things right. Diarrhoea is the body's way of getting rid of toxins and germs, so let the stomach work through the problem itself for a day or two and help the body to cleanse itself naturally. Don't panic or take strong anti-diarrhoea pills, as they will only interfere with the body's own system. It is an inconvenient thing, but stay at home and rest for a day or two following this simple regime.

General guidance

When your digestive system is upset you should be very cautious about what you eat. It doesn't matter if you eat nothing for a couple of days, but it is very important that you drink lots of water to replace all the lost fluid, otherwise you could become dehydrated, which is the primary problem with diarrhoea.

• Look at your tongue. In the initial stages it will be very moist and shiny, but with persistent dehydration it can become parched and often shrivelled. A light grey coating shows the entire digestive system is angry.
• Check your pulse (see pages 128–9). If the rate is over 90 per minute you are dehydrated.
• Look at your skin. Dehydrated skin loses its elasticity and looks lifeless.
• Check how much urine you passed. If you are dehydrated you will pass less.
• Drink at least 2 litres of fluids a day. To ring the changes from plain water try a herbal infusion (see page 147). If you become dehydrated you may also need to replenish lost salt.

Meal suggestions

Rice soup (congee)
Wash ½ cup of basmati rice thoroughly and add to 4–5 cups of fresh chicken stock or plain water. Add 1 tsp chopped root ginger, ¼ tsp ground turmeric (an antibacterial), 2 bay leaves,

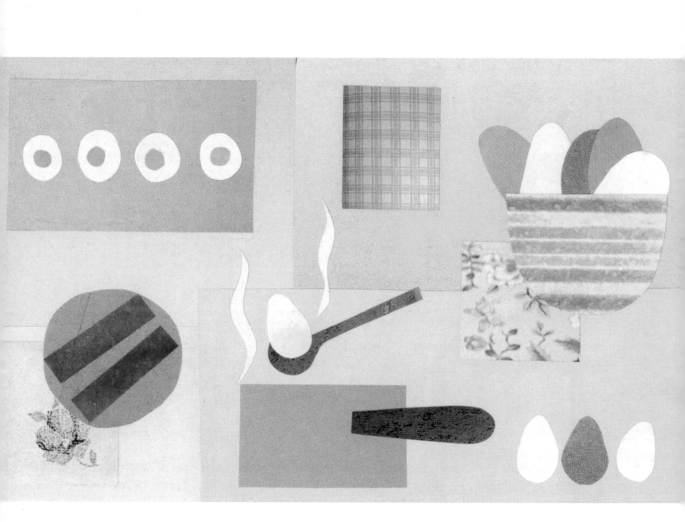

2 cardamom pods and a short length of cinnamon stick. These spices act as digestive stimulants. You can also add some chopped carrots and a little salt to taste. Simmer for 45 minutes, adding water if necessary and stirring to make it smooth. This is a thick soup and quite filling. (Take out the bay leaves, cardamom and cinnamon before eating.)

Kichri rice with yoghurt

Soak and rinse 1 cup of rice and 1 cup of yellow lentils (see page 73). Put the rice and lentils in a pot with 500 ml water, a cinnamon stick, 2–4 cardamom pods, 1 tbsp butter and ½ tsp salt. Boil until the water has nearly evaporated and then continue to cook on a low heat until the water has entirely gone. Shake the pot every now and then –

when the rice stops shifting the kichri is ready to be served with plain live yoghurt as a dressing or side dish. There may be a thin layer of rice sticking to the bottom of the pot – don't eat this.

Psyllium husks

1 tbsp of these stirred into a cup of live yoghurt will act as a binding agent. The yoghurt's bacteria will also help to overcome the pathogenic bacteria in the gut. Eat twice a day. (NB: these husks have the opposite effect if stirred into milk.)

Eggs

Boiled eggs (see illustration above) are binding as well. They help to slow down hyperactivity in the gut, and 6–8 eggs a day often has a settling effect.

Sip all teas slowly, both to enjoy the flavour and to allow your tastebuds to identify the taste. Avoid drinking it too hot, as very hot liquid will irritate the stomach lining. Try not to put milk in your herbal tea, as milk reduces the potency of the herbs and can clash with their taste.

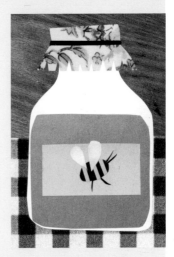

Indian tea Heat 2 cups of water in a small pot. As the water comes to the boil add 1 tsp Darjeeling or Assam tea and a small pinch of salt. Boil for 30 seconds then let it infuse for 2 minutes. Strain and drink, with or without the addition of a little warm milk (milk reduces its potency). You may add a little honey or brown sugar to taste, but preferably no more than 1 tsp. Make tea from good-quality leaves (two leaves and a bud makes the best tea), not the powdered waste put in tea bags.

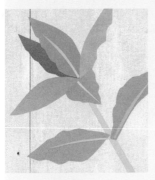

Mint tea Menthol has a soothing effect on the gut. Boil six fresh mint leaves in 2 cups of water for five minutes. Let them infuse for two minutes. Strain and add ½ tsp of honey. You can make mint-scented Indian tea by boiling the mint leaves first for 5 minutes and then the tea leaves as above. Do not add milk to this combination tea as this will absorb the essence of the mint.

Liquorice tea Liquorice has an anti-inflammatory property and soothes the gut. Boil liquorice sticks (1–2 per cup) for 5 minutes in water, cool and drink. It has a sweet aftertaste so no honey or sugar is needed.

Barley water For mild nourishment without straining the digestive system. Mix 1 tbsp of barley powder in a glass of hot water. Add 1 tsp of honey and a few drops of lemon for taste, as it is very bland. Drink three glasses a day.

Aniseed and basil tea Useful for mild stomach cramp and mucus discharge. Boil ½ tsp aniseed and 6 basil leaves in 2 cups of water for 3–4 minutes. Infuse for a couple of minutes, strain and drink. The aniseed will have a sweet aftertaste. Drink 2–3 times a day.

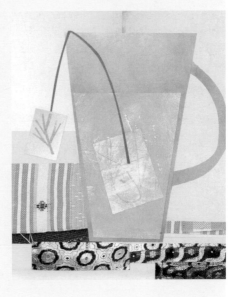

Pomegranate tea Pomegranate contains iron and cobalt, which has a stool-binding effect. Boil the skin of half a pomegranate in half a litre of water for 15–20 minutes. Cool for 30 minutes, then strain. Drink one cup with a little honey twice daily on an empty stomach.

a breath of fresh air

Although many people associate bad breath with the mouth (tooth and gum decay will make your breath smell bad), the embarrassing problem of halitosis originates further down. The distinctive odour of nail varnish on the breath, for instance, is caused by an excess of carbohydrates. If halitosis is a problem, my advice is to:

• Maintain good dental hygiene (see gingivitis, page 184).
• Reduce gut fermentation by avoiding yeast products.
• Eat fish and avoid meat, as putrefaction of protein can produce a strong smell.
• Avoid desserts and brush your teeth immediately after meals – sweets cause fermentation.
• Check you are drinking enough water (2 litres) in between meals.
• Use Neem Ayurvedic toothpaste (see page 220).

In traditional Persian and Arabic cultures, which the Moghuls brought into India, it was customary to sweeten the breath with a cup of rose, orange blossom, kewra or other floral essences in water. You can do the same thing after meals (see page 220).

INDIGESTION OR HEARTBURN

Discomfort and shooting pains just under the ribcage are the result of too much acid in the stomach. The excess acid regurgitates from the stomach up the oesophagus (foodpipe) and some of it can get sprayed into the bronchial tract, causing an intense burning sensation (heartburn) in the chest.

Dietary guidance

Avoid the following:
• Citrus fruit.
• White wine and champagne, beer and neat spirits.
• Nuts.
• Chillies or spicy food.
• Canned food and commercially bottled fruit containing citric acid as the main preservative.
• Vinegary foods.
• Taking medicines like steroids, painkillers or high doses of vitamin C (over 1000 mg).
• Drinking very hot liquids.

The following may help:
• Some vegetables and herbs have alkaloids that neutralise stomach acid. These often have a bitter taste that many people don't like, but try aniseed and chives added to dishes. Ayurvedic medicine recommends bitter gourd, fenugreek and drumsticks (a kind of stringy Indian pod), which are all bitter vegetables.
• Try mashed potatoes with 1 tsp each of aniseed and freshly chopped chives stirred in. If you are hungry, steamed or poached fish or chicken as an accompaniment is easy on the digestion.
• As an alternative to taking antacids when the heartburn starts, sip ice-cold milk or take a pinch of salt in a cup of strong mint tea (cooled) (see page 147).

Other beneficial suggestions

• Eat slowly (wolfing down your food can bring on indigestion in the first place).

• A walk after eating will encourage the digestive process and help avert indigestion.

DIVERTICULAR DISEASE

The colon, the final part of the digestive tract, is where the last nutritional elements of our food, such as calcium and magnesium, are absorbed and the waste waits to be eliminated as faeces. When the digestion is in good working order this happens smoothly and without delay, but pressures such as constipation and excess gas may cause sections of the intestine's lining to balloon. In time these stretched areas can form permanent sacs (diverticuli) where faecal matter accumulates. Sometimes the diverticuli are congenital. Someone with diverticuli may appear to be constipated – a swollen abdomen and no bowel movements – but when the full diverticuli suddenly overflow the stools may be very loose or liquid. This alternating sequence of constipation and diarrhoea, especially with a pattern of four days of constipation followed by two days of diarrhoea, often indicates diverticular disease. When diverticuli become infected (they make good breeding grounds for bacteria), the result is diverticulitis.

Dietary guidance

The best cure is prevention, but once diverticuli have formed, follow the guidelines for irritable bowel syndrome (pages 150–54). Plenty of fibre in your diet will help keep things moving in your intestines, but this should be soluble fibre, not insoluble types, like bran (see pages 13–14).

Gastric (peptic) ulcers

Pain on an empty stomach and shortly after eating is a characteristic symptom of a gastric ulcer. Normally, the mucus lining protects the stomach walls, but if this is damaged, then acid in the stomach can aggravate the gut wall to such an extent that it ulcerates. One of the causes of such damage is a bacterium, *Helicobacter pylori*, so antibiotics have been effective in treating both stomach and duodenal ulcers.

For my PHD project, the treatment of peptic ulcers with acupuncture, fifty patients were put on a standard ulcer diet and also received fifteen sessions of acupuncture. The results were astonishing – 68 per cent had their ulcers healed within six weeks without using drugs to reduce stomach acid. They were all pain-free and symptomless. (The study continued for twelve months.)

I am therefore convinced that the best advice for gastric ulcers is to avoid acidic food and drinks (see pages 40–41), combined with a course of acupuncture.

Irritable bowel syndrome is usually defined by the following symptoms, which may or may not appear together: diarrhoea, constipation, bloating in the stomach, heartburn, burping, flatulence, abdominal cramp or distension and rumbling in the abdomen. In other words, if you have any digestive problem that does not have an identified cause (food intolerance; bacterial, viral, parasite or fungal infections; diverticulitis; auto-immune disorders; hereditary or genetic defects etc.) then it is diagnosed as IBS. Doctors are baffled by this condition and, because diarrhoea of unknown origin is the key factor, they think that stress is the main cause, which is why some prescribe antidepressants.

Over the past two decades I have closely interviewed, observed and treated patients with these symptoms, drawing my own conclusions. First, I considered the most common symptoms:

diarrhoea and constipation
Generally, IBS is characterised by soft gassy stools or diarrhoea with occasional abdominal cramps

(diarrhoea being the more common feature of IBS have led doctors to the notion that the bowels are irritated). Constipation can be accompanied by symptoms that are linked with IBS (abdominal discomfort, flatulence and so on), but it is not brought about by an 'irritated bowel' – indeed, it is irritants, in the form of purgatives, that are used to stimulate the bowel and relieve constipation. Alternating constipation and diarrhoea may indicate diverticulitis (see page 149).

abdominal pain
There are two main types of abdominal pain: intermittent and continuous. Intermittent pains are caused by spasms of the intestinal walls, but continuous pain (lasting for several hours at a time) can have a number of causes, including ulcers or fissures anywhere in the intestinal tract, inflammation of the appendix, knotting of the intestines or a tumour. However, many people suffer from this sort of continuous pain that cannot be tracked down to a specific cause. The source remained a mystery to me until I studied

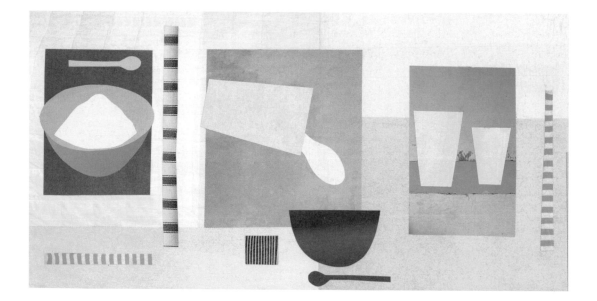

the muscles, tendons and fatty layer of the abdominal wall. Injured ligaments (constant bloating and stretching of the abdominal walls by gas), small herniations into weak spots in the abdomen caused by overlapping muscles, and inflamed fatty lumps on the abdominal wall from weight loss will all cause just this type of indefinable pain.

bloating

This is usually due either to swallowing air while eating fast or the reaction of acidic gastric juices leaking into the alkaline environment of the duodenum. If the bloating occurs an hour or so after eating, then this chemical reaction is the cause. If the bloated feeling happens almost immediately after eating, then the most likely cause is swallowed air in the stomach. If one bloats a couple of hours after a meal and has a lot of flatulence, then the likely cause is gut fermentation due to yeast or candida overgrowth, especially if the feeling is associated with extreme fatigue and a heady sensation 2–3 hours after eating as gas and toxic alcohols are produced and absorbed in the gut.

hiatus hernia

Sometimes excessive gas in the abdominal region and high stomach acid levels may cause hiatus hernia. This is a condition in which the pressure of abdominal air pushes the stomach wall up through the diaphragm into the thoracic cavity. The pain is acute and will last until the entrapped stomach wall is released. The pain moves up to the breastbone, back and even into the neck. Such pain also causes great distress because it is so close to the heart and many sufferers have believed they were having a heart attack.

My experience and observations have led me to find that IBS, rather than having no definable causes, has in fact multiple causes, a multifactorial condition like chronic fatigue syndrome, psoriasis or cancer. The following factors play an important role in IBS:

food intolerance

Sensitivity to a certain food or foods can be congenital or acquired, and reactions vary both with time and from person to person (see pages 197–8).

overgrowth of candida or yeast in the gut

This is a highly controversial area of medicine, but in recent years some doctors are beginning to understand the role that these fungi play in some health problems. Bloating, abdominal cramps, extreme fatigue an hour after eating, diarrhoea, rumbling in the tummy and flatulence can all be the result of too much candida or yeast in the gut.

excess stomach acid (hyperacidity)

The digestive process requires both acidity (from the stomach's gastric juices) and alkalinity (from bile secreted by the liver, via the gall bladder). Because what we eat can increase the acidity of the stomach but not the amount of alkaline bile to neutralise it (see page 28), too much acid in the stomach upsets the balance that makes for comfortable digestion. The heartburn, stomach pain and bloating that excess stomach acid cause are very much part of IBS. Moreover, bile suppresses the growth of fungi in the gut, so a lack of it can permit the candida or yeast overgrowth described above. In short: more acid means that there is less bile available for intestinal digestion.

parasites and worms

There are numerous parasites that thrive in the gut, quite unharmed. They absorb nutrients from the gut and produce toxins, which may cause excess mucus secretions, flatulence, abdominal cramps and other symptoms. Some sensitive tests are now available to detect their presence, and eliminating them helps reduce or cure these symptoms.

Because IBS is a multifactorial condition and some of the causes are difficult to identify, people try different treatments aimed at just one cause. Without tackling all the contributory causes, this approach is unlikely to bring lasting relief. When the condition persists for a long time, it can make life a misery without ever being life-threatening. The whole day begins to focus on digestive problems and the proximity of a toilet. Long journeys, queues, concerts and theatrical performances, even crowds, all become situations to avoid. The fear of embarrassment becomes obsessive and sufferers lose confidence and the ability to enjoy themselves.

My approach is to:
• Avoid foodstuffs that may invoke intolerance.
• Improve digestive ability.
• Build up general energy.
• Restore confidence.
• Increase the willpower to stick to a long-term regime.

General guidance

Do not have:
• Foods and drinks that encourage abdominal gas (see flatulence, pages 144–5).
• Yeast and fermented products: bread (including pizza), soy sauce, yeast extract spread and beer.
• Sugar and sweets, which feed the yeast.
• Milk and cheese (milk, if tolerated, is alright in small amounts).
• Very spicy food.
• Too many nuts.
• Fried and greasy food, including rich, creamy sauces, as these disrupt digestion.
• Alcohol in excess, which affects the liver and slows bile secretion.
• Canned or commercially preserved food, because of the citric acid used as a preservative.
• Coffee, as it tenses up the gut and may cause constipation.

Make sure you:
• Eat slowly and chew well. This will help the tastebuds identify the food and send messages via the brain to the digestive system to supply the right mix of digestive juices for the type of food.
• Eat soft foods. These do not need the vigorous churning and breaking down of rough, hard foods, and the stomach can soon pass them through to the next stage of digestion.
• Drink fresh mint tea (see page 147). Taken with a little honey, this helps calm down the hypermobility of the intestines.
• Rest for a short while after lunch. As explained in Chapter 3, this is good practice for everybody, but is especially beneficial if you have digestive problems. If possible, lie for 10–15 minutes on your left side, and then 10–15 minutes on your right. Allow yourself longer after a heavy or fatty meal.
• Walk for 10–15 minutes after dinner in the evening, to encourage your digestive process to start up when it may not want to (see page 99).
• Follow your after-meal walk with a simple yoga position such as Valiant Posture or *Bajrasana* (see my book, *Therapeutic Yoga*, page 220) which helps the abdominal organs to get an extra supply of blood.
• Eat live yoghurt (see page 24 and illustration on page 150).

One of the treatments that makes a world of difference to IBS sufferers is relief from recurrent diarrhoea. This is not a total cure, but removing the embarrassment of rushing to the toilet and the constant fear of accidents is a huge morale booster. My recommendation is to follow the Diarrhoea-free Diet (opposite). This is a boring regime, but a monotonous diet means that the digestive system is not overloaded by having to cope with a variety of foods. A plain 'meat and potato' type of diet absorbs most of the fluids and so helps to form firmer stools, while avoiding roughage slows down the hypermobility of the intestines.

Helpful nutritional supplements

Because the short-term Diarrhoea-free Diet is

the Diarrhoea-free Diet to be followed for 6–8 weeks

ban from your diet:
- Bread and cereals.
- Fruit, vegetables and salads (except those specified below).
- Dairy products except cottage cheese and yoghurt.
- Coffee.
- Alcohol.
- Fizzy water.

breakfast
- 1 or 2 hard-boiled eggs with a pinch of salt or black pepper.
- 1 pot live yoghurt or 200 g cottage cheese with 1 tsp organic honey.

VEGETARIAN ALTERNATIVE:
- Porridge or oatmeal.
- Yoghurt or cottage cheese (as above).

lunch
- Marinated, grilled fish or chicken with mashed or boiled potatoes (without skins).
Before cooking the fish or chicken, pierce all over and smother with a mixture of 3–4 tbsp yoghurt, 1 tsp olive oil, ½ tsp garlic paste and ½ tsp salt. Leave to marinate for 2 hours or overnight.

  If you are at work, prepare the chicken or fish at home (it is just as good cold) and buy a jacket potato to eat with it. You can add a little olive oil and salt, but don't eat the potato skin.

VEGETARIAN/VEGAN ALTERNATIVE:
- Pasta with olive oil or the insides of a jacket potato with a little butter or oil and a pinch of salt.

dinner
- Chicken soup. Skin and chop in small pieces half a baby chicken (poussin) and put in a pot with 1 clove of garlic, 1 cinnamon stick and 750 ml water. Boil for 10 minutes and then simmer for another 20 minutes.
and/or
- Minced chicken or meat with digestive herbs. If using beef, pork or lamb, ensure it is very lean (less than 5 per cent fat). Put 200 g meat in a pot with 2 cloves of garlic (chopped), a thumb-sized piece of ginger (chopped), a pinch or two of black pepper, 6 fresh mint leaves (or ½ tsp dried) and 500 ml water. Bring to the boil, put the lid on and cook on a medium heat until the water has disappeared. Add 1 tbsp olive oil and gently stir the mince until it is slightly brown in colour. Add salt to taste.
or
- Grilled fish. Marinate fish steaks or fillets in an olive oil and garlic paste for 10–15 minutes. Grill, then remove the skin before eating.

  Eat your choice of the above with potatoes (mashed or boiled), boiled carrots, mushy peas, soft-cooked dahl or yellow lentils, or mushy rice.
Mushy rice Don't use an easy-cook rice. Soak 200 g of rice for 10–15 minutes then rinse thoroughly 4–6 times, using a spoon or your hands to stir as you wash it. Put in a pot with 1.5 litres of water (1 litre for basmati rice). Bring to the boil, cover and simmer until the water has disappeared and the rice is soft.

  If you are eating out, order grilled fish, chicken or steak, or roast lamb or beef, or game (including wild duck such as mallard) with potatoes (no skins), rice or pasta (no sauce apart from olive oil).
VEGETARIAN/VEGAN ALTERNATIVE:
- Kichri rice with yoghurt (see page 146), served with boiled carrots or stir-fried potatoes. (Vegans can omit the yoghurt or substitute soya yoghurt.) Boil 2–3 potatoes until just cooked. Cut each into 4 and fry in a little olive oil or butter until the potato pieces are light brown. Sprinkle some dried mint leaves over the potatoes halfway through frying. Add salt to taste.

through the day
- Keep up your fluid intake with about 2 litres of water. For a change, switch to weak tea or herbal infusions (see page 147).

afterwards
Gradually introduce variety into your diet. Start with cauliflower, broccoli (florets only), asparagus, swede, turnips, peas, soda bread and mild spices. Cautiously introduce one item per week. If there is a flare up, extend the stricter diet for another 2–3 months.

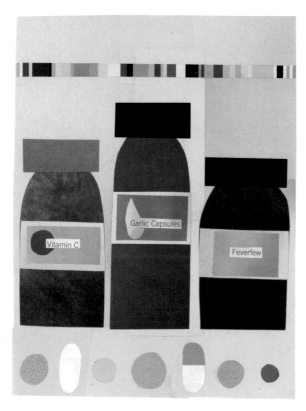

based on protein and complex carbohydrates and no roughage, you will need to take a multivitamin + mineral tablet every day to make up for the lack of fresh fruit and vegetables.

Vegetarians and vegans will find this diet particularly restricting. Supplement it daily with:
• Up to 10 almonds, soaked for 24 hours and skinned. Eat with honey and chew very well before swallowing.
• Proprietary protein powders (available from healthfood shops), taken in warm water with honey or molasses sugar twice a day.
• Daily general multivitamin + mineral capsule.

Other beneficial treatments

• Vigorous exercise increases the absorption of foods and nutrients in the intestines as the extra demands on the body pressurise it into seeking more nutrition. 'Tricking' your body in this way improves digestion and so will help to form stools.
• Yoga, for relaxation and to relieve stress.

Kidney stones

Kidney stones are accumulations of crystals and can be excruciatingly painful if they pass from the kidneys into the urinary tract. There are two types of crystal, and urinary analysis, via your doctor, will tell you whether your stones are formed of oxalates (derived from oxalic acid in onions, spinach, asparagus, tomatoes, kidney beans, brassicas etc.) or urates (derived from red meat, offal, cheese, shellfish etc.). This will tell you which types of food you should eat less of.

Plenty of water helps flush the kidneys, discouraging crystals from massing. Also try some of the following:
• Watermelon juice (2–3 glasses a day).
• Carrot and celery juice (1–2 glasses a day).
• Cucumber juice (2 glasses a day).
• Weak barley water (1 tbsp in 1 litre of water) with a little honey and a few drops of lemon juice for flavour (2–3 glasses a day).
• Fennel tea (3–4 glasses a day).
• Chickpea 'juice': wash ½ cup of black chickpeas and soak in 250 ml of water overnight. Drink the strained water first thing in the morning.

A frequent urge to go to the toilet and a burning sensation as you urinate, sometimes accompanied by pain in the lower abdomen, can indicate a urinary tract infection. A feeling of grit in the urinary tract and a slight fever can be additional symptoms. The usual medical response to this is a course of antibiotics. This is fine, but lingering and chronic problems of this nature are on the increase and the answer is not to continue various antibiotics for months on end.

Apart from general health – a rundown body will always be more open to infection – hygiene is the key here. Bacteria are not going to survive the kidneys' filtering system, so the source of infection is from the outside, not inside. As well as scrupulous personal hygiene, be aware that oral sex and, in men, prostatitis are common causes.

General dietary guidance

Avoid anything that will raise the acidity of urine and irritate the infected area:
• Citrus fruits.
• Pineapple.
• Dry nuts.
• Vinegar.
• Alcohol.
• Chillies and spicy food.
• Excess garlic.
• Painkillers and supplement tablets that contain citric acid.
• Canned sauces.
  Also avoid yeast and fungal foods that may encourage thrush, particularly if you have taken antibiotics. This includes:
• Cheese.
• Bread.
• Mushrooms.
• Beer.

Do not avoid drinking fluids because urination is painful. Plenty of water, at least 2 litres a day, will make things better not worse. Help neutralise the acidity of your urine with:
• Cranberry juice (with minimum sugar).
• 2–3 glasses of carrot juice a day.
• Mint tea made with fresh leaves (see page 147).
• 3–4 cups of chicken soup without vegetables (see page 153) a day.
• Fenugreek. Soak 1 tsp of seeds in a glass of water for 6 hours or overnight and drink on an empty stomach in the morning and evening. Fenugreek, being alkaline, acts as an antacid. For fenugreek recipes see page 157.

Other beneficial treatments

• Massage: regular massage to the neck and shoulders improves blood flow to the pituitary, helping to keep the immune system in good order. Massage in general also reduces stress – stress opens your body to infection and increases stomach acidity.

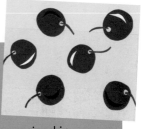

cranberries
Long appreciated for their high vitamin C content, cranberries have gained in popularity since their ability to combat urinary tract infection has been recognised. The berries stimulate the secretion of a chemical in the kidneys called lippuric acid, which prevents the adherence of bacteria on the urinary tract and so protects against infection. The arbutin in cranberries fights yeasts and so is useful in discouraging thrush and other yeast infections. Cranberries can also be used in poultices to treat wounds.

chapter 16
metabolic health

Our bodies run on a complex combination of interdependent electrical and chemical systems that, for the most part, react in synchronicity and keep themselves in balance in a truly amazing way. Sometimes, however, a malfunction occurs that causes an imbalance. There are rare enzyme deficiencies (usually from birth) that cause serious metabolic dysfunction, but more common are the disorders that arise when a body develops an inability to regulate levels of a particular enzyme or glandular secretion. What we eat plays a key role in controlling the effects of such over- or under-production, and in keeping to a minimum the potential harm such an imbalance can wreak on the body.

DIABETES

People with diabetes have an inability to control the amount of glucose (sugars) in their blood. Normally, blood sugar levels are managed by insulin, secreted by the pancreas. A failure to manufacture sufficient insulin and therefore metabolise sugars efficiently can be either a genetic problem (known as insulin-dependent or Type 1 diabetes) or brought on in later life (known variously as non-insulin-dependent, Type 2 or late-onset diabetes). The second form is becoming more and more common and, if not stemming from direct damage or infection to the pancreas, can be attributed in part to diet and a lack of exercise – it occurs more frequently among the overweight.

All diabetics need to control their diet carefully, and Type 2 diabetics, especially in the early stages, can often balance their blood sugar levels without resorting to medication. A sensible diabetic diet will also help guard against the complications of diabetes brought on by excess sugar molecules in the blood system. These can clog small capillaries, impairing circulation and leading to gangrene.

Another common side-effect is impotence. Clogging in the tiny capillaries in the eye can also affect vision (routine eye tests can pick up an early diagnosis of diabetes) and in the kidneys lead to their shrinkage and malfunction.

Dietary guidance

The first step is to get your sugar levels down. Once your blood glucose is within reasonable bounds, you can allow yourself some leeway – you will get to know your own tolerances. At all stages, take advice from a qualified dietitian or health professional and get your blood sugar levels checked regularly.

To begin with, as well as banning all the obvious sugary foods such as cakes and sweets, I recommend you stop eating:
• Honey.
• Fruit.
• Sugar-rich vegetables such as parsnips, carrots and beetroot.
• Alcohol.

recipes to stabilise blood sugar levels

The following recipes all help to control the release of sugar into the bloodstream. However, avoid potato dishes on a regular basis; once a week is about right.

crispy pancakes

Mix enough warm water into cornflour or chickpea flour to make a soft dough. Add salt to taste. Break off pieces and form into small balls. Roll out each ball into a thin circle. Heat a little butter in a frying pan (not so hot that it burns and colours), and cook each pancake gently on one side and then the other. These pancakes go well with yoghurt.

potatoes with fenugreek

2–3 medium potatoes, diced
2 tablespoons olive oil
400 g fenugreek leaves or 100 g dried
½ teaspoon turmeric
a pinch of paprika (for colour and mild
  spicy taste)
salt

1 Fry the potatoes in the oil, keeping them moving about the pan. Add the fenugreek and keep stirring.

2 Add the spices and a pinch of salt, cover and cook on a gentle heat for 15 minutes, stirring from time to time to stop them sticking (sprinkle with a little water if the moisture from the potatoes is insufficient).

fenugreek chicken

1 large onion, chopped
2 cloves garlic, chopped
2 tablespoons olive oil
2 chicken breasts, diced
1 tablespoon fenugreek seeds,
  soaked overnight or 400 g
  fenugreek leaves (sold as methi
  in Indian shops)
salt
black pepper

1 Quickly fry the onion and garlic in the oil.

2 Add the chicken and fenugreek (drain the seeds), salt and pepper to taste. Stir thoroughly, sprinkle with a little water, cover and cook on a low heat for about 20 minutes, stirring regularly to stop it from sticking.

The body converts starchy carbohydrates into sugars, so you must also avoid:

• Bread.
• Pasta.
• Potatoes.
• Cereals.
• Ordinary flour and rice (but see below).

If you need to lose weight you may also have to reduce your fat intake.

Menu ideas

Breakfast
• Boiled or poached eggs.
• Cottage cheese or unsweetened yoghurt.
• Spelt bread (made from seeds).
• Beansprouts (see page 52).
• Pancakes or unleavened bread made from cornflour or chickpea flour (see page 157).

Main meals
To begin with these will be predominantly protein and vegetables: plenty of fish and lean meat with green vegetables and pulses. Here are some ideas:
• Incorporate chives into a green salad – these help to control sugar absorption in the gut. Enliven the salad with a dressing of plain yoghurt spiked with a little black pepper, salt and a pinch of cumin.
• Reduce the starch in rice to an acceptable level with extra washing and rinsing. Soak 1 cup of rice in water for 30 minutes. Wash thoroughly. Add 10 cups of fresh water and boil rice for 20 minutes. Pour off the remaining water (which will be cloudy with starch). Add 4 cups of boiling water and boil for a further 2 minutes. Strain into a sieve and pour over more boiling water to rinse off more starch. This rice will not taste like ordinary rice and may be a bit chewy because of the protein, but it makes a good accompaniment to a main dish with a sauce.
• Fenugreek controls sugar absorption in the intestines. It has an individual, slightly bitter taste, but is useful for diabetics (see page 157).

Snacks between meals
Too little glucose is potentially as dangerous to a diabetic as too much, so to keep blood sugar levels steady, do not go too long without something to eat. Long gaps without food will cause your blood sugar to drop (hypoglycaemia), leading to dizziness and, if not remedied, hypoglycaemic coma. Again, you will come to know the rhythm and tolerances of your own body and to take into account extra glucose used up in exercise. The following foods make great snacks for diabetics:
• Fresh fruit (dried has too great a concentration of sugars).
• Oat biscuits or rice cakes.
• Corn on the cob.
• Crispbread with hummus, cottage cheese or taramasalata.
• Vegetable broth.
• Raw vegetable batons with low-fat dips.

Helpful nutritional supplements

• Bitter gourd. This is a traditional counter-measure for diabetes. It prevents the absorption of sugars in the intestine and it is also said that the alkaloids it contains facilitate the synthesis of glucoproteins in the liver which helps control blood sugar. It is a powerful antacid and the bitterness suppresses the appetite. If you are able to buy these members of the squash family (in ethnic shops and markets), try them as a juice or side dish.

To make bitter gourd juice (see illustration opposite), wash and chop 4–6 bitter gourds and run the pieces through a juicer; add a dash of salt. Drink it twice a day about 15–30 minutes before a meal – it is very bitter and has an aftertaste, so pinch your nostrils and drink it straight down. Many patients who have persevered with this find it has helped them get their diabetes under control.

To serve bitter gourd as a vegetable, chop 4–6 medium-sized gourds and 1 large onion and fry in a little olive oil for 5 minutes. Add salt and black pepper to taste, then cover and simmer for

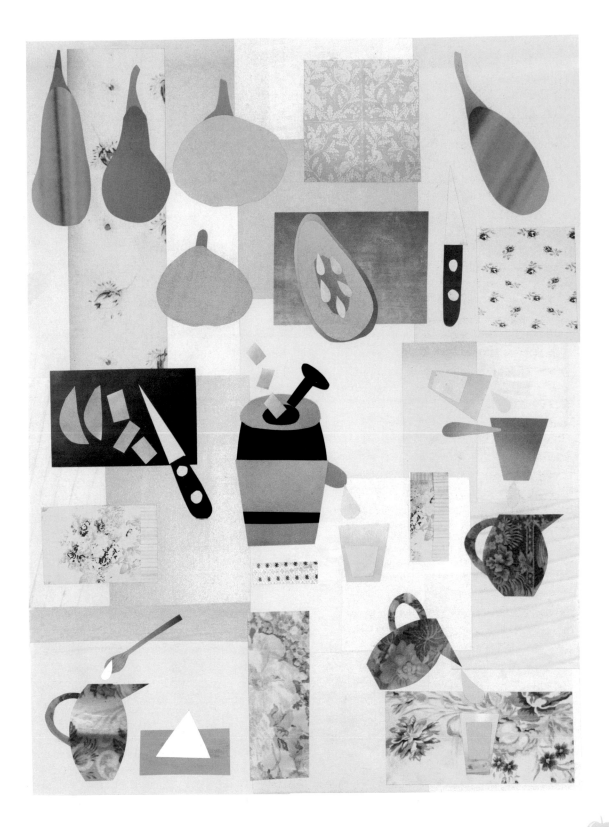

10 minutes, stirring from time to time. Sprinkle with a little water and simmer for a further 10–15 minutes (the gourds' skins take time to soften).

Other beneficial treatments

• Exercise is important in keeping blood vessels clear of accumulating sugar molecules. Brisk walking, therapeutic yoga, light weights and swimming are good exercises that not only improve the metabolic rate but also maintain good circulation.
• Massage aids circulation, especially to parts of the body prone to diabetic arthritis or circulatory complications: hip joints, hands and feet, neck and spine. It also helps sciatic pain because glucose molecules can block small blood vessels feeding the nerves, which can especially aggravate large nerves like the sciatic. A twice-weekly massage to the neck and shoulders will aid blood flow to the brain. More blood means more glucose is supplied to the pituitary-hypothalamus area, satisfying the appetite centre and therefore reducing the craving for sugar. I have observed in thousands of my patients how reducing sugar and carbohydrate cravings makes diabetic control much easier.

> Brisk walking, therapeutic yoga, light weights and swimming are good exercises that not only improve the metabolic rate but also maintain good circulation.

GOUT AND METABOLIC ARTHRITIS

As we digest and absorb what we eat, one of the by-products of protein is uric acid, which is usually eliminated through the kidneys. If your body is not metabolising protein efficiently, uric acid can instead get deposited as crystals on the inner surface of the joints, especially toes, ankles and knees. This causes acute inflammation, making the affected joint extremely painful, red, swollen and stiff.

General guidance

Gout is very much affected by diet. Once the acute phase is overcome, then a sensible low-protein diet will keep it at bay.

When the condition is acute and painful, conventional physicians usually give anti-inflammatory drugs and something to facilitate the elimination of uric acid through the kidneys. A simple but effective measure, however, is to fast for a couple of days. Allow your body to rest and take nothing but water (see Chapter 6). This gives the body a complete rest from anything that might aggravate the inflammation. The body then deals with the crystals naturally and the inflammation subsides. (Do not fast for longer than this, as fasting for more than three days sometimes causes the breakdown of fat and muscles, and uric acid levels can go up and increase the symptoms of gout.) If you are unable to fast, then begin the diet opposite straight away. A mild anti-inflammatory drug may be necessary to relieve the pain until the build-up of uric acid crystals has dispersed.

Follow a short fast with a week or two on the following diet, to allow your body to settle down completely:

• Avoid all animal proteins, including eggs and dairy products.
• Follow the Regimen Therapy (see chapter 7) for other foods to avoid.
• Drink fresh carrot, celery and ginger juice, which helps reduce inflammation and acts as a diuretic.
• Drink nettle tea as a diuretic.
• Use turmeric in cooking, as it has good anti-inflammatory properties.
• Drink at least 2 litres of water a day to flush the system.
    Thereafter, limit your intake of or avoid completely:
• Red meat.

• Alcohol.
• Shellfish.
• Offal.
• Cheese.
• Citrus fruits.
• Coffee.
• Limit your salt intake and keep drinking plenty of water.

Other beneficial treatments

• Rest as much as possible to avoid exacerbating the throbbing pain in the affected joint.

THYROID PROBLEMS

The thyroid gland secretes a hormone, thyroxine, which affects our metabolism. The amount of thyroxine that is produced depends on the level of stimulation from the pituitary gland, the state of the actual glandular tissue (an auto-immune disorder can cause the body's own antibodies to attack the thyroid) and sufficient iodine, the main element of thyroxine.

    Too much thyroxine (hyperthyroidism) increases the metabolic rate, causing you to feel very hot and your heart to beat more quickly, which results in palpitations, hyperactivity and weight loss (through burning off fat however much you eat).

    An underactive thyroid, predictably, has the opposite effect and in uncommon, severe cases can markedly slow the brain's function or development.

Dietary guidance

Nutrition can play a useful role in helping to counter a malfunctioning thyroid.

When the thyroid is in overdrive:
• A low-roughage, high-protein diet is useful.
• Avoid excess salt, coffee and alcohol altogether as these will just add fuel to the fire.

For an underactive thyroid:
• Cut down carbohydrates to one meal a day, and rely on porridge, potatoes, pasta and rice, avoiding sugar, sweets, alcohol and bread.
• Eat iodine-rich foods such as seaweed, aubergine and jamun (an Indian berry).
• A diet similar to the one recommended for diabetics (see pages 156–60) may help to keep the weight under control.

Nutrition can play a useful role in helping to counter a malfunctioning thyroid.

chapter 17
respiratory health

Every time we breathe in we are supplying our body with the oxygen it needs to survive, and every time we breathe out we are expelling carbon dioxide and waste products (such as excess alcohol, ketones and nitrous gases). Just having a stuffy nose for a couple of days has a debilitating effect: a headache from the build-up of mucus in the sinuses and a general lassitude from the extra effort of trying to breathe and the reduction in oxygen reaching our muscles. Included here, alongside actual infections of the respiratory system, are illnesses that have the effect of inhibiting our breathing, such as colds and flu.

COLDS

Such great technological advances have been made that it is said that a surgeon based in London can remove the gall bladder of a patient in Sydney through telemedicine. Yet medical science has not been able to find a cure for the common cold. We know it is viral in origin, so antibiotics are of no use. It is said that if you treat a cold it will be gone in a week, and if you don't it will go in seven days. The best thing we can do is give the body as much help as possible in curing itself.

The most important fact behind a cold is that the virus will lodge and proliferate in a body that is run down. Often it follows on the heels of catching a chill by exposure to cold air, air-conditioning or getting wet (especially in the head) in cold weather. The body expends a lot of energy in compensating for this acute loss of inner heat and the immune system becomes vulnerable. Opportunistic viruses, present in abundance in the atmosphere, then try to enter the body through the nasal passage where they begin to thrive. The body's defensive reaction is to 'wash' out the

The best thing we can do is give the body as much help as possible in curing itself.

multiplying virus with floods of nasal mucus and sneezing – a classic example of the body's sanogenetic powers wrestling a pathogenic force (the virus). In most cases the body wins and we get off with sniffles and sneezes. If the body loses, the virus penetrates deeper, inflaming the throat, sinuses and lungs.

If a cold is treated as soon as it starts, then the secondary complications are unlikely to set in. It is not a bad thing to be attacked by a cold virus every now and again – it makes you pay attention to your body rather than take it for granted.

recipes to soothe a cold

Ginger and black pepper tea
Boil a few slices of fresh root ginger and a pinch of ground black pepper in water for 4–5 minutes. Add a few drops of lemon juice and a little honey.

Anti-cold soup
Peel and chop some onion, leek, potato, garlic and root ginger. Boil these in water or home-made stock for 20–25 minutes. Stir in a little ready-made mustard, black pepper and salt to taste and a few drops of lemon juice. Drink twice a day. It will warm your body (you may break out in a sweat), which will inhibit the multiplying of the virus.

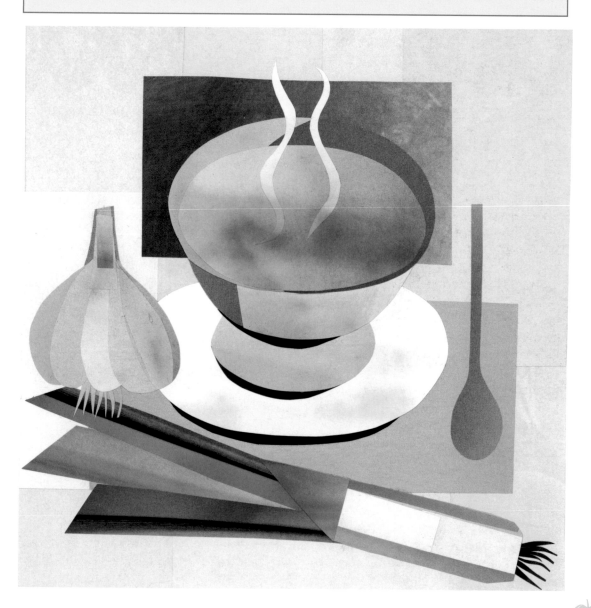

Dietary guidance

Avoid:
• Very cold food and liquids: chilled drinks, ice cubes or ice cream.
• Dairy products (which increase mucus production).
• Mushrooms and cheese (fungi also increase mucus production).
• Foods that put pressure on the digestive system such as rich and creamy sauces and fried foods.

Drink the following:
• Plenty of warm fluids – a teaspoonful of brandy with honey in a cup of warm water is great at bedtime.

Helpful nutritional supplements

Vitamin C: take 500 mg 2–3 times a day for five days.

Other beneficial treatments

Using nasal sprays or antihistamines to stop a runny nose may be convenient, but it is not a good idea – all they do is constrict the blood vessels to stop fluid filtering through them. Instead, try the following:
• Sinus oil nasal drops. Mix small quantities of 1 part sesame oil, 1 part mustard oil and 2 parts sweet almond oil. Put one drop of the mixture in each nostril and sniff up. Do this twice a day. Mustard is a powerful antibacterial and possibly has some antiviral properties.
• Nasal douche. For this you will need a neti pot (used in yoga) or an old-fashioned inhaler. Dissolve ½ tsp of table salt in a glass of lukewarm water and pour the saline mixture into the inhaler. Tilt your head to the left, open your mouth wide and breathe through your mouth. Insert the nozzle into your right nostril and slowly pour in some of the water. Concentrate on breathing through your mouth and the water will come out of your left nostril. Repeat the procedure with the other nostril while tilting in the opposite direction. This will help the body to wash away the virus.
• Homeopathy. Try Ferrum Phos, Aconite 30 or Gelsemium 30. Take two tablets three times a day for three days.

SINUSITIS AND CATARRH

These are both effects of an over-production of mucus. This can be a reaction to a cold or flu virus, to an infection anywhere in the head (such as earache or tooth decay) or a chronic condition related to a food intolerance or working in a polluted environment. Chronic constipation also causes excess mucus discharge in the sinuses as the body tries to eliminate toxins.

Mucus build-up in the sinus cavities can be quite painful. Press the two points above your nose where your eyebrows begin (or in line with the inner corners of your eyes if you have very bushy eyebrows that meet in the middle) – if it hurts your sinuses are probably blocked.

Dietary Guidance

Avoid:
• Foods that encourage mucus, e.g. dairy products.
• Fungal foods, such as mushrooms and cheese, and vegetarian meat substitutes made with fungi.

Every day:
• Drink fresh apple, carrot and ginger juice, plus plenty of water (but avoid very cold drinks, which can make the sinuses hurt more).

Other beneficial treatments

• Try sinus oil nasal drops and douche (see above).

Influenza, like a cold, is a viral infection and, again like the cold, has many mutations which makes it difficult to build up a natural immunity. The best we can do is to be as healthy as possible so that our bodies are in good condition to fight off the infection without succumbing to the worst aspects of it.

Many people call a bad cold the flu, but the viruses are different. Some of the symptoms are the same because the virus enters through the nose and the body's first response is to fight back with an abundance of mucus to flush it out. If the virus gets past these defences the next stage is a sore throat, often accompanied by earache, headaches and the typical flu symptoms of immense fatigue and muscle ache, shivering and fever. If the infection spreads down to the lungs there will be copious amounts of mucus (again, the body's defence mechanism) coughed up as phlegm, and inflammation of the bronchial tubes.

It is not by chance that flu viruses seem to be most prevalent with the onset of winter and again in the spring. When the weather turns cold viruses seek a warm host in which to survive and multiply – and humans are ideal winter homes. Early spring is when our bodies are most likely to be run down. We are probably eating fewer good-quality fresh fruit and vegetables, as by this time many have been in long-term storage or grown unseasonably in hothouses (see Seasonal Foods, page 47). We may also be exhausted from the effects of over-indulgence and stress from Christmas or other winter revelries.

The conventional doctor's advice for flu is bed rest, plenty of fluids, vitamins for vigour and paracetamol for fever. The integrated medical approach is very much along the same lines.

Dietary guidance

Restrict yourself to soups and water or herbal teas to spare the digestive system from having to work hard when all the body's energy needs to be concentrating on fighting infection. This is the reason for bed rest too – sleep as much as you can. Don't force children to eat if they don't want to.

Drink plenty of water, but at room temperature or warmer (cold water may aggravate a sore throat and very chilled water is mucus-producing).

Treatment of fever

The fever that characterises flu is the body's way of killing the virus. The virus thrives at the normal body temperature of 37°C, but if the body heat rises to around 38°C the virus cannot multiply. Higher temperatures, around 40°C, begin to affect the brain and make you delirious, so the ideal is to curb the worst of the fever but without inhibiting the body's natural weapon. At 39°C use cold packs or fans to cool the room, or small doses of paracetamol if necessary. If your temperature rises any higher, use paracetamol and don't hesitate to call in a professional if your temperature doesn't drop back to between 38°C and 39°C.

Helpful nutritional supplements

• To boost your immune system take 500 mg of vitamin C and a B-complex tablet 2 or 3 times a day; 15 mg of zinc can also be helpful in fighting infection.
• Ginseng in tea or capsule form.
• Chawanprash, an Ayurvedic tonic of some two dozen herbs and minerals (available from the Integrated Medicine Centre, see page 220).

Other beneficial treatments

• Massage, especially around the neck, shoulders and spine.
• Sinus oil nasal drops (see opposite).
• Homeopathy. A number of homeopathic remedies are ideal for flu.

Ginger and liquorice tea

Boil a thumb-sized piece of root ginger (chopped), 2 peppercorns and 2 liquorice sticks in 2 cups of water for 5 minutes. Strain and add a pinch of baking soda and a little honey. Drink this at least three times a day, sipping slowly. The baking soda helps soothe an aching body and sore throat, the liquorice has some antiviral properties and the ginger will tone you up and make you sweat.

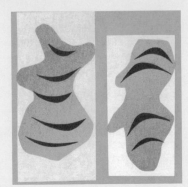

Spicy soup

This soup is nutritious enough to be satisfying but light enough to be easy on the digestion. Eat the chicken only if you feel hungry enough. The spices will make you sweat, which is a natural way of cooling the body and eliminating toxins.

Put the chicken in a pot with 1½ litres of water. Bring to the boil and simmer for 45–60 minutes to get a good stock. Add the vegetables and spices and simmer for a further 20–30 minutes. Non-meat eaters can make the same soup without chicken.

1 poussin or small chicken chopped into small pieces
2 cloves garlic, chopped
1 thumb-sized piece root ginger, peeled and chopped
10 peppercorns
2 medium onions, finely sliced
1 potato, diced
1 cinnamon stick
5 cloves
4 bay leaves

Energy juice

This delicious drink contains the vitamins, minerals and enzymes the body needs in distress. The herbs calm the mind and reduce anxiety. If the ingredients are stored in the fridge, take them out an hour or so beforehand so that the juice is not too cold. Drink the juice mid-morning or mid-afternoon.

6 carrots, peeled
2 apples, peeled
a thumb-sized piece of root ginger
10 basil or mint leaves

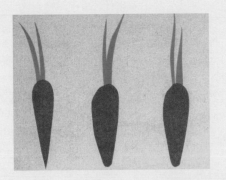

Place all the ingredients in a food processor or juicer and blend until smooth.

These are both infections of the lungs, often brought on by a cold or flu virus that has not been stopped by the body's natural defences or where the lungs are already under strain, such as in someone with asthma. As we have seen, the body tries to flush out the infection with a stream of mucus. However, accumulations of excess mucus that remain in the body can also become breeding grounds for bacteria – it is bacteria that turns phlegm yellow or green. Pneumonia causes one or both lungs (double pneumonia) to become inflamed and is usually accompanied by fever and a feeling of constriction that makes breathing painful. The dry, ticklish cough that is often an annoying part of the infection is due to spasm of the bronchial tract, like asthma.

Dietary guidance

All the information on preventing a cold or flu from taking hold applies here – bronchitis is a common complication of both. Warming foods are all helpful:

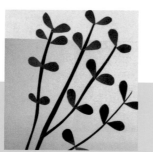

thyme

The aromatic oils extracted from thyme, thymol and carvacol, have antibacterial and antifungal properties, good for cuts. Thymol is used as a mouthwash and is a good expectorant of phlegm. It relaxes smooth muscles and is therefore helpful for bronchial and asthmatic coughs. Thyme also relieves intestinal and menstrual cramps.

• Chicken broth with added black pepper, ginger, drops of lemon and onion, drunk two or three times a day.
• Stir-fried vegetables with grated ginger, mustard paste, garlic and fenugreek leaves (add sliced potatoes or peas to tone down the bitter taste of the fenugreek).
• Lentil soup cooked in lamb broth, spiced with garlic, ginger and coriander.
• Carrot and ginger juices, but store the carrots at room temperature – cold carrots will produce cold juice (see opposite).

Helpful nutritional supplements

• Multivitamins with zinc – 15 mg a day.
• Ayurvedic chawanprash or bioprash, 1 tbsp a day (see page 220).
• Buttercup syrup.
• Certain herbs help to expectorate mucus. For example, Dr Ali's winter tea (see page 220) contains liquorice and fennel. Drink 2–3 cups a day. After taking an expectorant you should follow it with a mucus-drying preparation: mix 1 tsp of ginger powder with 1 tsp of honey and take it twice a day to help dry up the mucus.

Other beneficial suggestions

• Avoid smoking or being in a smoky atmosphere, which can be a major irritant to sensitive lungs and cause bronchitis to become a chronic condition.
• Inhalation with peppermint balm or a vapour rub helps to soothe a ticklish cough.
• Visiting a sauna (dry heat) or even two or three days in a hot, dry climate helps to cure a persistent ticklish cough that remains after you have recovered from the main ailments.
• Yogic breathing exercises are very effective for bronchitis, especially the cleansing breath described in my book *Therapeutic Yoga* (see page 220).
• Neck and spine massage.

chapter 18
bone and muscle health

Everyone knows that nutrition and exercise are needed to keep muscles in good shape, but it is easy to forget that bones need nutrition and exercise, too, as do our joints and the ligaments, tendons and cartilages associated with them. Regular exercise that doesn't overstrain muscles and joints will help prevent many problems in later life.

Protein builds up muscle and provides energy to exercise (sumo wrestlers eat up to 3 kg of meat a day to maintain their muscle bulk and tone). Many of the foods high in protein – eggs, meat, fish, dairy products – also contain calcium and vitamin D (see page 16 for an explanation of their relationship), which are essential for bone and muscle health. Muscles of all types, which includes the heart, cannot function without calcium, and if they do not have a steady supply of this mineral they will 'steal' from the bones, which become weak and brittle.

Muscles also need B complex vitamins and potassium and magnesium to aid with contraction and relaxation (see pages 17 and 21 for good sources of these vitamins and minerals).

Foods that are not conducive to bone and muscle health include:
• Caffeine, which tenses muscles and prevents them relaxing.
• An excess of acidic foods (see pages 40–41) can cause inflammation of the ligaments and joints – in traditional Indian medicine acid foods such as vinegar, lemons and oranges are banned from regular use as a preventative measure.
• Excess red meat and fatty foods, which cause arthritic changes in the joints.
• Refined sugar, which also causes arthritic change. Diabetics are often prone to joint pain because of their difficulty in regulating the amount of sugar in their blood.

The two main chronic disorders of the bones and their connective tissues are osteoporosis and the various forms of arthritis. Osteoporosis, a weakness or brittleness of the bones most usually found in older people and especially women is covered on page 111.

Arthritis means inflammation of the joints. Joints are made up of bone surfaces coated by a layer of cartilage. Usually it is this cartilage and the synovial membrane covering the joint surface that gets inflamed, producing fluid that accumulates in the joint space. The result is swelling, stiffness and pain in the joint, sometimes also redness and a sensation of heat. There are several types of arthritis, of which the most widely encountered is **osteoarthritis**, caused by wear and tear or degenerative changes in the joint surface. This is the typical arthritis due to ageing. A variation on this is **traumatic arthritis**, when the cartilage is destroyed by an accident or joint fracture (such as a sports injury). **Rheumatoid arthritis** is quite different, a painful condition caused by auto-immune changes in the body (see page 171). There is also **metabolic arthritis**, brought on by a metabolic imbalance such as diabetes or gout (see Chapter 16); **infective arthritis**, caused by an infection of the cartilage; and **psoriatic arthritis**, a complication of psoriasis. These last two are rare.

Joint replacement is becoming ever more sophisticated and often vastly improves the quality of life when the chance of self-repair is remote, as in rheumatoid arthritis or severe osteoarthritis in the elderly. However, prevention is always better than cure, and it is worth doing everything you can by way of diet and exercise to delay the onset of osteoarthritis and to minimise its effects. If you are due to have surgery on your joints, see page 213.

This 'wear and tear' form of arthritis is a common complaint among the over-60s and most usually occurs in the knees, hips, spine and finger joints. Typically, it involves stiffness in the joints in the morning, which wears off as the day goes by, periodic swelling and occasional clicking noises from the arthritic joints. It can be extremely painful and can make everyday movements such as going up and down stairs very difficult at times.

Dietary guidance

Avoid all:
• Acid foods. The synovial membrane, which lines the joints, acts in some fashion as an excretory organ, hence the build-up of crystals of uric acid that cause such pain in gout. An excess of acid can also lead to crystal formation, so it's best to limit your intake of tomatoes, strawberries and raspberries as well as the more obvious citrus fruits and vinegary products. Cider vinegar with honey is often recommended for osteoarthritis, but I cannot agree that this is helpful.
• Sugar and all derivatives, including alcohol. Sugar and alcohol increase joint stiffness.
• Dairy products. These increase mucus production and may increase fluid secretion into the joints.
• Canned and preserved products. Chemical preservatives will irritate the joint surfaces.
• Yeast (see pages 44–5).
• Excess red meat, offal, shellfish or anchovies. Too much of these foods can cause a build-up of uric acid.
• Ice-cold water/ice cubes. These make joints sensitive.
• Foods that cause a lot of gas, such as pulses, mushrooms, radishes, cucumber and fizzy drinks. The link between flatulence and joint pain is a curious one, but a phenomenon that has long been observed. My own possible explanation, based on logic, is that abdominal gas causes compression of the dorsal aorta, the main artery of the lower half of the body. This artery is separated from the abdominal cavity by just the peritoneum enclosing the abdominal organs. As gas expands the intestines, pressure increases on the front and rear of the abdomen. In front the belly swells up, but at the back pressure builds on the dorsal artery, causing sluggishness of the circulation in the entire body as resistance to the blood flow increases. This may cause joints to ache.

Instead eat:
• Garlic. Improves elimination of gas from the abdomen (see above) and has mild anti-inflammatory properties.
• Ginger. A mild anti-inflammatory; it also improves general circulation.
• Fenugreek. As well as anti-inflammatory properties, it is a diuretic and therefore removes the swellings in the body and improves morning stiffness. Soak 1 tsp of seeds in a glass of water overnight and drink the water first thing in the morning.
• Papaya and guava (see illustration on page 170). These fruits have mild laxative properties. They help eliminate toxins and gas from the body and therefore bring relief.
• Custard apple. A particularly good fruit for arthritis because of its anti-inflammatory and gas-relieving properties.

A weekly one-day fast is very beneficial. If overeating or excess consumption of the wrong things has caused the joints to react, a two- or three-day fast can relieve the pain and stiffness. Limit yourself to water or juices of fresh vegetables and non-citrus fruits. Afterwards the body feels relieved of its stiffness. See Chapter 6 for further advice on fasting.

A calcium-rich stock for non-vegetarians
Simmer meat bones for 1–2 hours over a gentle heat to get a stock enriched with gelatine and calcium. Use it as the basis for soups.

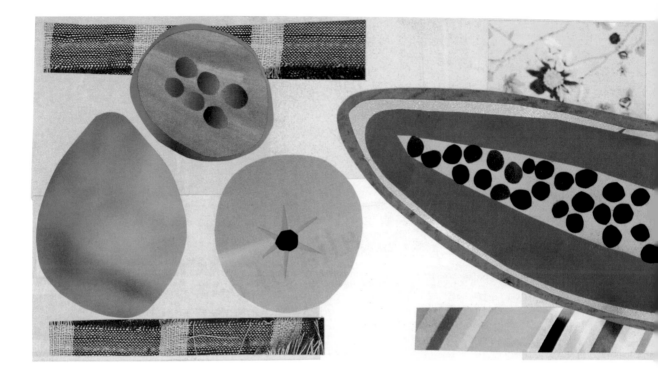

Helpful nutritional supplements

• Turmeric capsules, devil's claw, chondritin, MSM and glucosamine – all available over the counter – have anti-inflammatory properties and help repair joints.
• Haldi, an Ayurvedic supplement containing turmeric and other ingredients that help the joints (see page 220).
• Calcium. Arthritis is particularly common in vegetarians or the elderly, where lack of calcium may be a problem. This lack can also cause damaged joints to heal badly. Calcium is available in milk, but dairy products are not good for arthritis, so I recommend coral. Medicinal coral is specially collected and sold in sachets as coral calcium. Soak these as advised on the packet (usually 1–2 sachets in 1½ litres of water) and drink throughout the day. Do not open the sachets, as the rough particles can irritate the stomach. The body seems to absorb calcium in this form better than as tablets or capsules.

Conventional medicines

Where there is severe inflammation and pain, a brief course of non-steroidal anti-inflammatory drugs and painkillers can be helpful in buying time to give the body a chance to respond to the other measures mentioned above. Once arthritis becomes chronic, these drugs are of no use, and have their own side effects.

Other beneficial treatments

• Massage with Dr Ali's Arthritis Oil (see page 220). Concentrate on the affected joints and the muscles above and below the joints.
• Physiotherapy and exercise help arthritis to some degree but do not give full relief, although there are yoga exercises that can help (see my book, *Therapeutic Yoga*, page 220).

This is a progressive degenerative disease that occurs when the body's auto-immune system goes awry. Somehow the body develops a sensitivity towards its own connective tissues and cartilages and tries to reject them, causing inflammation and deformity. This type of arthritis is more common in younger people and often leads to crippling disability as the cartilage on joints gets destroyed. (NB This is not the same as rheumatism, a relatively rare disease that is triggered by certain bacteria affecting the heart and then the joints. When people complain of 'rheumatism' or 'rheumatics' it is usually osteoarthritis.)

Dietary guidance

Follow the guidelines for osteoarthritis on page 169.

Conventional medicines

In severe cases, steroids in very low doses can be the only way to slow down the degenerative process, especially if there is no opportunity to carry out *panchkarma* (see below). Sometimes immuno-suppressants and chemotherapy are used to counteract the destruction wrought by the patient's own antibodies, but the price is very heavy. The toxins affect the liver, kidneys and the whole body, so it is better if possible to take advantage of simpler methods of treatment.

Other beneficial treatments

• *Panchkarma* is a complete Ayurvedic programme of five cleansings (*panch* = five). It involves a strict vegetarian diet (often just rice, vegetables and lentils); body massage; nasal douche with oils; enemas using medicated oils or emesis (vomiting – rarely used); and head massage with oil. It is believed that oil removes the toxins from the body, which makes it an effective cure for ailments like rheumatoid arthritis. I strongly recommend

massage of the head and body for this type of arthritis. The oil is massaged into the body with the hands, and herbal poultices are used to impregnate the deeper layers of the skin. When the poultice is scraped off, it brings with it whatever toxins the oil may have absorbed. The massage improves circulation and the medicated oils have anti-inflammatory properties. The head massage helps blood flow to the brain (underneath the scalp is a rich network of veins). Improved cerebral circulation helps the pituitary gland to function better and so the auto-immune reaction is corrected through the hormonal system.

• Acupuncture relieves pain and stiffness and, combined with the Regimen Therapy (see chapter 7), has helped many people.
• Homeopathy.
• Oil massage and Ayurvedic oil bath (see page 220).
• Gentle exercise is beneficial, but this is a very painful condition that should not be exacerbated by vigorous movement.

muscular cramp

Cramp from excessive exercising is caused either by an accumulation of lactic acid (relieved by massage or rest) or dehydration – for which the answer, of course, is to drink plenty of water.

Dehydration can also cause muscles to go into spasm at night, but the more usual reason is calcium deficiency and potassium imbalance (which can be brought about by taking a diuretic regularly). Muscles need calcium to contract, but when there is a deficiency they like to shut down and go into cramp, or, in other words, become non-functional.

Coral calcium (see page 170) can be taken as a supplement if you are deficient, but a more likely cause of cramp is the poor absorption of calcium. Avoid getting constipated, as this impairs calcium absorption through the colon (see page 140).

heart and circulatory health

Circulating reliably and constantly without any conscious effort on our part, blood supplies nutrients and oxygen to every part of our bodies. Any upset in this system has repercussions on our health, and if oxygen fails to reach our brains for even a short time the result is irreparably damaging and soon fatal.

The two key elements of circulation are the heart, which is the system's pump, and the arteries, which channel the blood to every part of the body. The veins play a more passive role, providing a return route to the heart for the 'spent' blood. Problems occur either when the blood cannot flow freely at the right pressure through the arteries or when the heart's pumping action is altered or impeded.

The problems associated with blood pressure and the heart cannot be totally resolved by what we eat, particularly in the advanced stages, but a regime of healthy living – diet, exercise and stress management – makes the biggest contribution to warding off trouble. The advice in the first two parts of this book is all about preventing trouble; what follows is for those who already have problems with either blood pressure or their heart – the two usually go hand in hand.

HIGH BLOOD PRESSURE

Two things will raise the pressure under which blood races through the arteries. The first is if the heart pumps faster, and the second is if the arteries themselves become narrower, forcing the blood (which stays at the same volume) through under greater pressure.

When we exercise vigorously we can all feel our heartbeat increasing, and then slowing down again as we rest. Such a temporary rise is normal. But other things can cause the heart to pump faster: hormonal secretions, including oestrogen (which is why high blood pressure has to be watched for in pregnancy and when taking oestrogen-based contraceptive pills) and adrenaline (increased by stress); illness such as fever; caffeine; excess salt; and some drugs. The heart does not so easily return to a resting rate from these, and high blood pressure – also known as hypertension – can become the status quo.

What can restrict the flow of blood through the arteries and raise blood pressure? Sudden rises are usually brought on by stress, which causes the kidneys to secrete angiotensin, which in turn causes the blood vessels to constrict. Usually of greater concern is the slow 'furring up' of the inner walls of the arteries with fatty plaque (just like limescale in water pipes). As well as narrowing the area through which the blood flows, these fatty deposits harden and make it more difficult for arteries to relax and dilate. They can also break off and form dangerous clots, or build up to such an extent that the pressure causes small blood vessels to block completely or rupture. Depending on where in the body this happens, the result might be a brain haemorrhage or stroke, kidney damage, loss of sight or heart failure. And the source of the fatty deposits that begin this descent into calamity is our diet.

High blood pressure is usually associated with ageing, and there is a natural rise in blood pressure after about the age of 60, but more and more people much younger than this are suffering from it.

A tendency towards high blood pressure can be genetic. If your family is inclined to hypertension, treat this as a warning sign that you need to take extra preventative measures early in life. See Your Health MOT (chapter 14) for information on checking your blood pressure.

Dietary guidance

Avoid foods that stimulate the heart into working too hard, such as:
• Coffee.*
• Too much ginger,* garlic, chillies and very spicy food.
• Salted and cured fish and meat.
• Red meat, including sausages.
• Shellfish.
• Crisps.
• Sweets and chocolate.*
• Preservatives (in most canned food).
• Processed foods.
• High-proof or excess alcohol.
Those marked * also constrict the blood vessels, as do salt and monosodium glutamate (MSG).

You should also avoid nicotine, cholesterol and excess sugar, which all lead to hardened arteries.

Foods that help include:
• Celery.
• Fennel.
• Herbal teas such as chamomile, fennel, nettle and dandelion.
These dilate the blood vessels in the kidneys, increasing their filtration capacity of blood.

Don't cut down your fluid intake, but encourage elimination of excess fluid in the body with mild diuretics such as:
• Carrot juice.
• Celery juice.
• Nettle tea.

Rethink your style of eating
Animal fats are the main source of cholesterol (see pages 14–16). A vegetarian diet with, say, fish once a week, will quickly control high blood pressure.
• Avoid fats and oils in cooking, even olive oil. This will reduce cholesterol intake and help weight loss.
• Heavy foods add to the tension in the body, so aim for lighter meals, especially in the evening.
• A day of fasting once a week is highly

deep vein thrombosis
A blood clot or thrombus in a vein can develop, most usually in the legs, from long periods of immobility, and is exacerbated under pressure, which is why it has become an issue on long-haul flights. The biggest threat from deep vein thrombosis (DVT) can come some time after it has formed. If it comes adrift and moves through the blood system to the heart or lungs it can cause a potentially fatal blockage (a coronary or pulmonary embolism).

The standard advice on long flights is to exercise regularly, not to cross your legs (which restricts the blood flow) and to take a small dose of aspirin, which thins the blood and makes it less

prone to clotting. While this is all helpful advice, the likelihood of blood forming clots in the first place has a more basic cause. The liver regulates most of the clotting factors in the blood and poorly oxygenated blood will develop cobweb-like fibres in which blood cells get trapped. An unhealthy liver (see pages 29 and 43) means your blood is not going to be in good shape either.

Help prevent clots by following the regime for high blood pressure (see above), and avoid nicotine and caffeine, which both constrict the blood vessels. Obesity and lack of regular exercise (not just walking up and down on long plane journeys) can also lead to thrombosis.

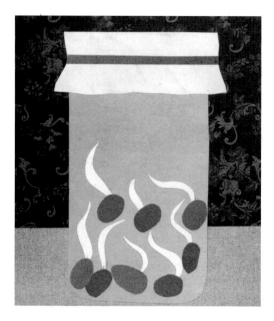

recommended (see Chapter 6). Regular fasting automatically reduces your overall salt and cholesterol intake, and helps with weight control, all of which is good for blood pressure. If you feel too hungry, make vegetable soup for dinner. (Cabbage, celery, carrots, peas and leeks are all good, but not potatoes. Add a little black pepper for extra flavour, but no salt – and make sure the stock you use is salt-free too.)

A semi-fast on another day is also beneficial: limit your food to a variety of fruit (except citrus fruit) and vegetable soup throughout the day.

Overweight people are inclined to have high blood pressure. The steps above will all encourage a natural weight reduction, but read also Chapter 14.

Remedial action

If you are already suffering the effects of chronic high blood pressure, I recommend the following Fat-free Diet, which can even help people who have genetically high cholesterol.

For at least three months, completely ban:
• All fats and oils. Dairy products (other than low-fat milk), oils (including olive oil), red meat and chicken skin are all out, as are most nuts, which have a high oil content.

• Alcohol.
• Coffee.
• Salt (if necessary for taste, use low-sodium or magnesium salt).
• Preserved foods, and all prepared sauces or meals, because you cannot truly gauge their fat and salt content.

You should eat:
Breakfast
• Selection of non-citrus fruit (you can have the occasional tangerine or other sweet variation, but eat the pith and fibres to counteract the acidity).
• Boiled egg white and/or cottage cheese with a little honey or crushed nuts.
• Sprouted beans or alfalfa (see pages 52 and 88 and illustration, left).
• Porridge or oatmeal with very low-fat milk or home-made cottage cheese (milk curds).

To make your own cottage cheese, bring 1–1½ litres of milk to the boil, then take off the heat. Squeeze in lemon juice drop by drop until the milk curdles. This will cause the casein, the curds, to settle at the bottom and the watery whey to remain on top. Strain off the whey (which contains some minerals and is often quite pleasant to drink when cooled if not too much lemon juice has been added). Rinse the curds gently with water to wash away any excess lemon.

This is a very nutritious, high-protein but low-fat food. You can have it with cereal or eat it on its own with a little honey or some crushed nuts on top.

Lunch and dinner
Make meal combinations with:
• Very lean meat such as skinless chicken or turkey breast, rabbit or veal.
• Fish.
• Vegetables.
• Rice.
• Lentils and pulses.
• Non-citrus fruits with a high vitamin C content, such as kiwi fruit, berry fruits, blackcurrants and

mango. Vitamin C acts as an antioxidant that helps to prevent plaque formation.

Because fats and oils are banned, except for what is contained within the meat or fish, your principal methods of cooking will be grilling, steaming and boiling. Occasionally you can use low-fat yoghurt as a marinade. You can't use salt, or much ginger or garlic, but do not shy away from making the most of other herbs and spices as flavourings – use all the thyme, rosemary, sage, parsley, coriander, cumin, turmeric, black pepper, tarragon, coriander and so on that you like. Use your imagination and make it as tasty as you can. Experiment with innovative ideas for soups, which are filling, and try new vegetables.

To begin with you may be irked by the lack of variety, but remember you are eating to fight something that is dangerous to your health and even life-threatening. A restricted diet may be the best thing you could do to save your health.

After three months on the diet, go for a cardiac check-up and cholesterol tests. If your blood pressure and cholesterol levels have dropped satisfactorily, continue on the same basic diet, but allow yourself to relax the rules a bit for two or three days a week. If not, stay on the strict diet. Keep having tests every three months, returning to the strict diet if your levels rise again, until you come to an optimum level. This may take a year. Continue to get your levels checked out regularly.

Conventional medicines

When blood pressure is very high, and complementary and traditional methods of treatment fail to bring about any long-term effect, then conventional medical drugs should be used. Some people at risk due to familial history, or people whose obesity, high-stress job or lack of discipline prevent their benefiting from the guidelines above are better off taking conventional medical drugs.

The drugs used to control blood pressure have the following basic functions:

• To slow down the heart rate (beta-blockers).
• To dilate arterial walls.
• To induce calm (tranquillisers).
• To reduce the volume of blood by increasing urine output (diuretics).
• To block blood-pressure-raising hormones in the kidneys.
• To inhibit the transmission of impulses to arterial walls and therefore prevent their constriction.

But keeping blood pressure 'under control' with drugs does not guarantee that complications will not set in, and the chances of complications are very high without a drastic and realistic change in the regimen of diet and exercise.

Helpful nutritional supplements

• Indian herbal medicines: Sarpgandha (*Rawolfia serpentina*) dilates blood vessels; jata mansi (valerian) slows the heart rate and also dilates arteries; shankh puspi is a tranquilliser; and gokhru is a diuretic.

Other beneficial treatments

• Exercise is vital. Begin slowly and steadily, increasing as your state of health improves. Avoid competitive sports such as tennis (unless you always win!), as the pressure to beat your opponent and frustration at losing are not conducive to lowering blood pressure. Walking and swimming are good.
• Yoga. Excellent for reducing stress, slowing the heart rate and relaxing muscles.
• Massage. To aid relaxation of the muscles and the mind, so lowering blood pressure. Deep-tissue massage can sometimes alleviate a sudden headache, tensed muscles and palpitations brought on by an acute surge in blood pressure.
• Acupuncture. Very effective for treating early stages of hypertension.
• Homeopathy. Also useful in the early stages.

So much is heard about high blood pressure that it is easy to think that low blood pressure can only be a good thing. But too low a pressure makes you feel lethargic and cold all the time. It can also lead to a poor appetite and a tendency towards constipation, a lowered libido and sometimes depression.

A sluggish circulation means poor blood flow to the brain, which can result in tinnitus (ringing in the ears), blurred vision, a craving for sugar, headaches, frequent yawning, mood swings, propensity to infections etc.

Low pressure is usually taken as below 100/60, although this may be a normal, healthy reading for some – a predisposition to low blood pressure can be genetic, and very fit people will also have a low reading when at rest. If you feel wobbly – and perhaps need to lie down – after a soak in a hot bath, you may have low blood pressure (as muscles relax and blood vessels dilate to reduce body heat in a hot bath, blood pressure drops).

Poor appetite, diarrhoea, fasting, heavy menstruation, depression, anaemia and hormonal imbalances such as thyroid or oestrogen deficiency can all cause blood pressure to drop and should be checked out by a professional, but the most common causes are a lack of protein or a poor diet generally.

Dietary guidance

The first thing to do if you have low blood pressure is to raise your protein intake. The moment you do this the chances are your blood volume will increase. Eat more eggs, fish and meat, including red meat. Other helpful foods and drinks are:

- Honey.
- Ginger.
- Garlic.
- Ginseng tea.
- Pomegranate.
- Spinach.
- Aubergine.
- Ginkgo biloba.
- Caviar.
- Brandy (a tablespoonful in a glass of water with a teaspoonful of honey).

You can also increase your salt intake, but avoid caffeine. It may seem like a pick-me-up because it constricts the blood vessels and increases the heart rate, but the effect is only temporary and is followed by a greater slump.

Other beneficial treatments

- Exercise is important. Concentrate on vigorous exercise like brisk walks, aerobic work-outs and swimming.

Our staying alive is reliant on our heart doing its job, for which, because it is a muscle, it needs a regular supply of oxygen-carrying blood. When restricted arteries (see high blood pressure, pages 172–5) decrease the blood supply to the heart the condition is known as **ischaemia**. Any increased effort, perhaps even going upstairs, demands more oxygen than the blood can supply, so the heart aches, just as leg muscles ache from running too much. This pain is called **angina**.

The failure of the heart to pump efficiently leads to circulatory problems, such as the accumulation of fluid in the legs or lungs. Pieces of the plaque that builds up in arteries can also break away and cause blockages that can interfere with the blood supply. If the blood supply is cut off completely to part of the heart by a clot, the heart cannot pump and you have a heart attack.

The heart can also be in danger of failing if it is put under constant strain. Very high blood pressure makes the heart beat fast which, over time, builds up the heart's muscles and enlarges the left side of the heart. An over-large heart risks not receiving enough oxygen. Obesity, similarly, puts extra demands on the heart with which it may be unable to cope, especially as the body's bulk probably makes exercise difficult.

Heart disease is one of the major killers in the West – yet it is largely preventable. The things that increase the risk are well-known and well-publicised: stress, lack of exercise, high blood pressure, diabetes, smoking, alcohol abuse… and the wrong diet. Heart disease has a strong genetic factor, so lifestyle plays a vital part in reducing the risk of dying prematurely from heart failure. Muscle-building drugs have caused enlarged hearts and heart failure in recent times – young sports enthusiasts should be very cautious.

Conventional medicine has made great advances in the treatment of heart disease and I think these should be used in preference to traditional medicine. Fortunately, heart muscles can repair themselves and function even though scar tissue is formed where the muscles have been damaged but – and I cannot stress this too strongly – the best medicine is avoiding trouble in the first place!

Dietary guidance

If you are suffering from ischaemic heart disease or are otherwise at risk, impose a strict dietary regime for a year or two:
Avoid:
• Fats and excess oils. Beware particularly of dairy produce, including cheese (but excepting yoghurt); red meat and high-fat meats like ham and foie gras; and fried and oily food, including stir-fries in Chinese restaurants, which are often cooked with lard.
• Coffee if you have high blood pressure (it constricts the blood vessels).

herbs for the heart
If you are on a low-sodium diet, make full use of herbs to add flavour to your meals instead of salt. The following herbs have therapeutic properties that are particularly beneficial for your heart and circulation:
• Garlic (lowers cholesterol).
• Basil (tones up the heart muscles).
• Chamomile (relaxes the mind).
• Fenugreek (lowers cholesterol).

• Excess salt (increases blood pressure). Watch out for foods that may be unexpectedly high in salt, such as canned or preserved foods; gravy powder and ready-made sauces; cured meats.
• Alcohol (helps absorption of fats).
• Chocolates, cakes and sweets (fat and sugar promote weight gain).

See also the Fat-free Diet described on page 174, which you could follow for a year, just getting the fats you need from fish and lean meat.

Cutting the things above from your diet does not mean it should be boring. Look out for new varieties of fish, fruit and vegetables. Expand your range of lean meat with guinea fowl, quail and game. Collect recipes for pulses from Asia, Africa and the Caribbean.

Vitamin C is also believed to be beneficial (its role in producing noradrenaline, which helps control blood flow, may account for this). It is also an antioxidant and helps prevent plaque formation in arteries. Take vitamin C in food rather than as a supplement. People often think that citrus fruits are the best source of vitamin C, but they aren't in fact the richest in the vitamin; what's more, they can be too acidic for optimum health (see page 41). Choose sweet varieties that will be less acidic, and eat the whole fruit, not just the juice. Other foods particularly high in vitamin C include:
• Raw sweet peppers.
• Chillies.
• Brassicas (the cabbage family), when lightly cooked.
• Kiwi fruit.

• Papaya.
• Strawberries.
• Blackcurrants.
• Rhubarb.
• Amla.

Amla, also sometimes called Indian gooseberry, is available in Ayurvedic outlets. It has the richest source of vitamin C of any plant – 20 times more than that found in an orange. The vitamin C is chemically 'bound' in such a way that it does not get easily destroyed.

A strict diet along these lines should allow your heart and arteries to improve to a state when you can then follow a more relaxed, varied diet, along the principles outlined in the Regimen Therapy (see chapter 7).

Fasting is also extremely helpful for keeping in check all the dietary factors that promote heart disease; moreover it helps to lower blood pressure and encourages a sense of calm, which relieves stress. Fast one day a week and, if possible, do a three-day fast every six months (see Chapter 6).

Other helpful treatments

• Yoga: this is stress-relieving and a good form of exercise without strain.
• Walking and t'ai chi are also recommended.

parsley
This herb is quite high in a number of vitamins and minerals, but is not usually eaten in sufficient quantity to contribute much to our diet in this way. However, it has long been used as a diuretic and can help to treat water retention and urinary problems such as cystitis. It improves blood circulation, and helps in labour as it stimulates contractions.

Heart disease is one of the major killers in the West – yet it is largely preventable.

varicose veins
These enlarged purple-blue veins which most commonly occur on the legs are caused by damage to a vein's valve, impeding the free flow of blood. Blood collects temporarily behind the valve, stretching the vein walls until, in time, they stay enlarged.

Some people are more susceptible to varicose veins than others. Venal veins are damaged by pressure, which is why pregnancy and a lot of standing (particularly if you are overweight) can be a trigger. Constipation can provide just this sort of pressure, so eat plenty of fibrous fruit and vegetables such as figs, papaya and brassicas, including beetroot, to stave off any sluggishness in the bowels (see Constipation, pages 140–44).

Gentle massage of the affected area helps, as can support stockings (available for men too, although women are more inclined to develop varicose veins). Avoid too much standing around as well.

Red blood cells contain haemoglobin and transport vital oxygen around the body. Blood with a haemoglobin content slightly below par is a common condition, especially among women, and particularly teenage girls. Haemoglobin has two components. Haem, the nucleus, contains iron and cobalt; these are what give blood its red colour, and anaemic blood actually looks less red. Globulin, the second component, is a protein.

Anaemia is caused by a deficiency of iron in the diet, or a poor ability to absorb it. As iron is absorbed by the stomach, inflammation of the stomach lining, gastritis caused by excess acid secretion or a stomach operation can all result in poor absorption. A strict vegan diet with little protein can lead to a deficiency in globulin, as can poor absorption of protein due to anorexia, cancer, severe IBS with diarrhoea or Crohn's disease.

Dietary guidance

Avoid spicy and sour food:
• Citrus fruits (in excess they can cause gastritis).
• Pineapple.
• Rhubarb.
• Vinegar.
• White wine and champagne.
• Canned products and tinned soups (which use citric acid as a preservative).

Eat foods high in iron, such as:
• Red meat.
• Spinach and other dark green leafy vegetables.
• Liver and offal.
  Also eat:
• Pomegranates (high in cobalt).

If you have plenty of iron in your diet and yet suffer from anaemia, the problem may be absorption. For those with recurrent gastric problems or diarrhoea, see chapter 15.

You should limit your consumption of tea, coffee and colas, which inhibit absorption.

Vegetarians need to ensure that they accompany iron from non-animal sources with vitamin C, to help absorption, and that they are getting sufficient protein.

Helpful nutritional supplement

• An iron supplement, taken over a short period.

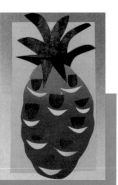

pineapples

Eaten in moderation, pineapple is a very therapeutic food. It contains an enzyme (bromelain) that tenderises meat, which makes it a useful digestive. Bromelain can also lessen blood's ability to clot, therefore helping to prevent deep vein thrombosis, heart attacks, stroke and so on, although it also increases a tendency to bruising. It eases constipation, treats jaundice (by improving liver function) and is effective against parasites and worms. Pineapple is a good source of vitamin C (like lemons and limes, it was a saviour in bygone days for warding off scurvy, and sought after by long-distance sailors in the tropics).

skin and teeth health

Our outer coverings – skin, hair and nails – are good indicators of our general state of health. They reflect the ageing process, react to stress and show up hormonal changes. If our skin goes dry and flaky, our nails grow ridges or our hair starts falling out unexpectedly, these are outward signs that all is not well inside. These parts of our body are also vulnerable to fungal infections. Whereas the immediate reaction is to treat a skin complaint directly with cream, traditional medicine regards skin problems as a sign of malfunction elsewhere in the body.

If the liver is malfunctioning, for instance, your skin will turn yellowish (jaundice), and liver and gut fermentation can cause seborrhoeic dermatitis. Allergies and food intolerances often show themselves in scaliness and itching. Calcium deficiency causes pale patches on the face and elsewhere, while excess stomach acid can make the skin extremely sensitive, so that simply bathing in hot water can cause a rash. Stress can also bring out rashes. All these indicate that the health of the skin is linked with the internal system.

Skin plays a major part in eliminating toxins from the body. The liver detoxifies the blood, and the kidneys then eliminate the toxins. The toxins of smaller molecular size will filtrate out of the kidneys, but the larger ones would get trapped in the blood unless the mucus-producing systems of the respiratory tract (nose, sinus) or the skin provided an alternative outlet. Eczema, seborrhoea, hydradenitis (inflammation of the sweat glands), urticaria, dermatitis and acne are the result of the excretory functions of the skin working overtime.

We may hate the look of various skin eruptions or rashes, but it is the body's own way of getting rid of the unwanted products or toxins. A weak or overworked liver will allow more toxins into the bloodstream that will have to be eliminated by the skin. A toxin-free diet will not only be better for you, it will give you a clear skin.

A quite different cause of skin complaints is an allergic reaction. Conditions such as eczema and hives are dealt with in Chapter 22.

The main problems of the teeth result from the build-up of plaque. This leads to receding gums, bone loss in the jaws and infection of the gums. All these problems are largely preventable with proper dental hygiene. Visit the dentist or dental hygienist regularly. Excessive grinding of the teeth at night, a symptom of stress, can weaken and damage teeth. Massaging the jaw muscles and the temples for a couple of minutes at bedtime can relax these muscles to prevent unnecessary grinding. A neck massage at bedtime can also help relieve this stress.

ACNE

Our bodies use several methods of eliminating unwanted matter, including via the skin. The sebaceous glands, just below the skin, secrete

fat-soluble toxins. If they are having to work overtime, the excess sebum they produce can irritate the subcutaneous layer of the skin, causing 'eruptions' in the form of spots and rashes.

Acne is a well-known bane of teenagers – one of the common side effects of the hormonal upheaval in these years is overactive sebaceous glands – but any body that needs to rid itself of excessive amounts of fat-soluble toxins can be troubled by acne, which is as likely to appear on the back or buttocks as the face.

Rashes and patches of red itchiness that appear anywhere where there are hair follicles may be due to the same overproduction of sebum that brings on acne. Known as **seborrhoeic dermatitis**, it can cause an angry red nose or whiteheads on the tip of the nose, an area particularly rich in sebaceous glands; it may also occur on a man's beard area, under the arms or on the scalp.

Dietary guidance

Keeping your intake down of foods that send the sebaceous glands into overdrive is going to help calm your skin at any age, even if hormones are the primary trigger. Avoid the following altogether for a month or six weeks, and then keep them within moderate bounds:
• Yeast and fungal products, which cause fermentation (and hence alcohol) in the gut (see pages 44–5). This means cutting out beer, mushrooms, bread, etc.
• Excess fat and salt, which are hard on the liver. So avoid fried food and crisps; sausages, cured meat and fish (bacon, smoked fish etc.); and cheese (except cottage cheese).
• Foods that make the skin sensitive, such as spicy foods and citrus fruits. These produce a lot of stomach acid, which is known to cause sensitive skin and joints. In homeopathy and traditional medicine, controlling stomach acid is essential for curing skin disease.
• Foods that tense up or constrict the blood vessels like highly spiced foods and caffeine (canned drinks as well as coffee).
• Chocolates and sweets (sugar encourages gut fermentation).

• Anything with a lot of additives.
• Shellfish (these are rich in uric acid, and some come from highly polluted seas).
• Cured and smoked meat and fish. These often attract bacteria and fungal spores present in the air which feed on the food's surface and produce toxic waste, which may then be excreted through the skin.
• Alcohol, which overworks the liver.

Have:
• Plenty of fluids to help your digestive system: 2 litres of water a day, and fresh fruit and vegetable juices – in place of citrus juices, try combinations of carrot, celery, apple and ginger.
• Organic foods whenever possible, to minimise the amount of undetectable toxins you are taking in; and make digestion easy by chewing well, eating slowly and following the other guidelines in Chapter 3.

Helpful nutritional supplements

• 500 mg of vitamin C per day.
• Bioliv, an Ayurvedic supplement (see page 220).
• Kadu (*Helleborus niger*), a detoxifying herbal tea. Soak 2 twigs in a cup of water overnight. Strain and drink in the morning.

Other beneficial suggestions

• Medicated skin creams, such as aloe propolis cream, will help relieve itching and inflammation. Dr Ali's Skin Oil (see page 220) is an Ayurvedic oil with natural antiseptic properties. In my opinion raw aloe vera pulp is the best natural product one can ever use. Those who have been treated on my India trips will vouch for it. Applied to the skin, the pulp removes itchiness and cures rashes of various types.
• Wash morning and evening with chickpea flour (known as gram or besoon in Asian shops). Make it into a paste with warm water, scrub your face with the paste and wash off with warm water. This removes a lot of the grease from the outer layer of the skin.
• Avoid smoking.

Dandruff and acne are often found together, because they have the same cause. Overactive sebaceous glands cause the outermost layer of skin, which is just dead cells, to flake off. On the scalp these flakes get caught up in the hair, and where patches of trapped flakes build up on the scalp, they create areas of frustrating itching.

Dietary guidance

Dandruff is made worse by alcohol and in particular drinks that contain yeast, such as beer.

Help control the activity of the sebaceous glands by giving them less work to do. Limit your intake of:
• Sugar and sugary foods.
• Fried and oily food.
• Cheese and butter.
• Very spicy food.
• Alcohol.
• Citrus fruits.
• Yeasty and fungal foods.

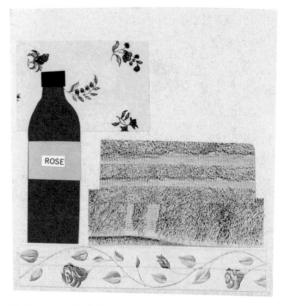

Other helpful treatments

• Scalp massage with Bioflame Ayurvedic scalp massage oil (see page 220 and illustration, above).
• A gentle anti-dandruff shampoo.

The encrusted, reddened skin that characterises psoriasis can become deep-seated and extremely painful. Elbows and knees are most frequently affected, as well as the scalp, where a crusty crown forms along the hairline. It can spread all over the body. The cause is unknown but there is always a history of severe shock preceding the first attack. The immune system seems to be involved, and recent medical treatment uses immuno-suppressants (those used in cancer therapy) to keep severe psoriasis in check, but at a heavy cost to the liver and kidneys.

As there is no actual cure the best treatment is to alleviate the aggravation and keep the skin as healthy as possible through diet. In conventional medicine the skin is only treated by topical creams, of which there are four types: antibiotic, antifungal, antihistamine (anti-allergic) and steroids (anti-allergic, immuno-suppressant). The few people I have helped were recommended a strict lifestyle programme to relieve symptoms and help the liver improve the condition of the skin.

Dietary guidance

Follow the dietary guidance for acne (see pages 180–81). It has been found that psoriasis sufferers can't metabolise vitamin D well, so exposure to sunshine often helps, as do foods rich in vitamin D, such as oily fish and breakfast cereals with added vitamin D.

Helpful nutritional supplements

• Kadu (*Helleborus niger*), a herbal tea. Soak 2 twigs in a cup of water overnight. Strain and drink in the morning.
• Ayurvedic tea.

Other beneficial treatments

• Soothing medicated skin creams, especially those containing aloe vera and propolis (see page 181).

• Baths in Dead Sea salts.
• Organic sesame oil to keep the skin soft.
• Bioflame oil (with oil of flame of the forest) and Bio Margosa shampoo with neem oil to help control the scalp encrustations (see page 220).
• Neck and spine massage to help blood flow to the pituitary gland, the main controller of the immune system.
• Relaxation and breathing exercises to help stress management.

MOUTH ULCERS

Painful little mouth ulcers can spring up without warning and are usually a signal that something is wrong somewhere further down the digestive system. This could be excess stomach acid refluxing back into the mouth, an inflammation or bacterial infection in the gut or a candida yeast infection. Mouth ulcers could also be a symptom of a lack of B vitamins – they sometimes occur following a course of antibiotics, which destroy the friendly bacteria in the gut that manufacture vitamin B.

Dietary guidance

To prevent ulcers from recurring:
• Stick to a two-day semi-fast on vegetable soup, fresh carrot juice and, of course, plenty of water. (See Chapter 6 for guidelines to successful fasting.) The vegetable soup recipe on page 57 can also be made with chicken or vegetable stock for this half-way fast.
• Follow a restricted diet for the next two weeks: eat only organic foods and cut out entirely foods and drinks containing yeast, sugar and excess acid (see Chapter 4).
• Build up the friendly bacteria in your gut, especially if you have been taking antibiotics. Eat live yoghurt (see page 24) and plenty of leafy green vegetables.
• Reintroduce other foods slowly, avoiding

obvious antagonists such as foods that are vinegary or otherwise acid, highly spiced or very salty.

To ease the soreness of an ulcer:
• Suck an ice cube.
• Use cloves to numb the area. Cloves are excellent anaesthetics. You can simply suck a clove two or three times a day until all its oil is extracted; gargle with water and a clove; or apply clove oil – stinging but effective.
• Avoid all acidic and highly salted food and drink.
• Eat melon, cucumber and other 'cool' foods (see pages 38–9) and avoid 'hot' foods such as red meat, chilli, garlic and excess spices.

Helpful nutritional supplements

• Make sure your bowels move well (if necessary, take 2 tbsp of psyllium husks in water at bedtime).
• 1 vitamin B complex capsule a day for a month.
• 1 acidophyllus and bifida capsule a day for a month.
• 2 twigs of kadu (*Helleborus niger*) soaked in a cup of water overnight. Strain and drink in the morning.
• Bioliv, an Ayurvedic supplement (see page 220).

Other beneficial treatments

• Homeopathy.

banishing gingivitis

This inflammatory gum disease is a major cause of bad breath, and infected gums can often produce pus. As well as careful oral hygiene and following the general dietary instructions for skin, the following regime should deal with the problem:

• 1 multivitamin + minerals tablet every day for three months.

• ½ tsp of table salt mixed into ½ tsp of pure mustard oil. Massage into the gums with your index finger gently for 1–2 minutes. Do this for a month at bedtime. Initially, pus will be sucked out by this mixture and then it will clear up. The mixture eliminates the germs and the gentle massage helps the gums to heal.

FUNGAL INFECTIONS

These are more common now than they used to be, because in general we have fewer 'good' bacteria in our bodies to keep them in check. Fungi often cause a problem at the fringes or openings of the body: hair, nails, mouth, vagina. While conventional antifungal preparations will kill them, and may be necessary for an acute infection, they will not ward off or give you any immunity against further attacks. Fungal infections can only be conquered by making the body strong enough to resist, so that fungi do not take hold.

The form that fungal infections take varies, depending on the location on the body:

• Nails. These become deformed and brittle; toenails are more often affected.

• Hair. Fungus attacks hair follicles, causing the hair to become weak and fall out. Alopecia is a form of fungal attack.

• Skin. Ringworm and tinea affect the skin. Other fungi can cause areas of depigmentation; most commonly caught by swimming in hot places.

• Feet. Athlete's foot is a type of tinea that causes peeling, itchy patches, especially between the toes.

• Vagina. Thrush (candidiasis) is relatively common in the vagina; for more information, see page 191.

Some fungal infections, such as alopecia and nail infections, are more difficult to treat than others, but all should be treated early when they first appear. The longer they remain on the body surface, the more powerful they become.

Dietary guidance

There are two principal steps to take. First, you need to avoid all foods that will lead to a proliferation of fungus (this includes foods containing yeast, foods high in sugar, as sugar feeds yeast, and fungal foods). This includes:

• Bread (including pizza and most flat breads).

• Beer.

• Yeast-extract spreads.

• Sweets and chocolate.

• Cakes.

• Dried fruit.

• Many ready-prepared sauces.

• Alcohol.

• Mushrooms.

• Cheeses matured with fungal growths, such as blue cheeses and soft cheeses with a rind.

• Foods that attract fungus to their surfaces, such as grapes, smoked fish and dried fruit.

Second, you need to build up your body's ability to fight off infection. To do this:

• Ensure that you are getting optimum nutrition from your diet, as described in Parts One and Two.

• Combine protein with vegetables and restrict carbohydrates to a minimum (eat a small amount of pasta, rice or potatoes, but combined with vegetables).

• A two- or three-day fast can be beneficial (see

Chapter 6), as can a vegetarian diet for about two weeks.
• Have a live yoghurt regularly to help build up 'friendly' bacteria (see page 24).

Helpful nutritional supplements

• Kadu (*Helleborus niger*). Soak 2–3 twigs in a cup of hot water and leave to soak overnight. Strain and drink in the morning. Repeat daily for 2–3 months.
• Capsules of caprylic acid or grape seed oil (consult physician).
• Infusions of vitamin C and B_{12} intravenously helps to boost the body.
• Acidophyllus with bifidus capsules.

Other beneficial treatments

For a fungal infection on the skin rub fresh lime juice on the affected area twice daily for 2–4 weeks (apply with cotton wool).

Massage of the neck and shoulders will help build up the body's own sanogenetic powers

For ringworm or skin infections in the groin area buy sulphur powder mixed with a 2 per cent salicylic acid-based cream and apply to the affected area once a day for a week
For athlete's foot use the following formula mixed in a bottle: 2 parts turpentine oil, 4 parts neem oil, 2 parts eucalyptus oil and 2 parts kolonji oil. Dowse a cotton wool ball with the oil and place it between the toes. Remove after 20 minutes and keep the area dry.
• Massage of the neck and shoulders, and yoga will help build up the body's own sanogenetic powers.

ROSACEA

Doctors are increasingly seeing this skin problem, which manifests itself as a very bright rose-red rash on the cheeks and the nose – often the shape looks like a butterfly, its wings spread out across the cheeks from the 'torso' of the nose. Sometimes acne-like eruptions on the tip of the nose exude a bright red sebum and are sore. Although the exact cause of this condition is not known, it is conventionally treated by strong antibiotics over a long period of time. I know someone who took tetracycline for over 20 years before he came to see me.

Dietary guidance

All the advice for keeping skin as healthy as possible (see acne, pages 180–81) apply here. Avoid alcohol and hot, spicy food, which can make the affected area more inflamed.

Helpful nutritional supplements

• Propolis/aloe vera skin cream as a calmant.
• Kadu tea (see above) and Bioliv (see page 220).

Other beneficial treatments

• Neck and shoulder massage. I give a lot of emphasis to this, as it helps the pituitary gland to boost the immune system. It has helped many patients. It seems likely that the hypothalamus (behind and above the pituitary), the higher centre for the autonomous nervous system, is involved in the manifestation of angry skin that characterises rosacea. The hypothalamus controls blushing in the exact area where the rosacea appears, and does get worse in hot conditions and during emotional states.

chapter 21
reproductive health

What we eat has a direct influence on our reproductive system, just as it does on the other functions of our body. It is well known that anorexia in teenage girls upsets or stops their periods, and that women who have been on low-fat, low-protein diets can experience trouble conceiving. But the right foods can also be a positive force: relieving painful menstrual and menopausal symptoms, improving sperm count and increasing fertility. Diet is also largely instrumental in controlling a complaint that is becoming more common: vaginal thrush.

PREMENSTRUAL SYNDROME

During the menstrual cycle, a woman's body comes under different stresses. Changes in her hormonal balance upset the normal equilibrium, as hormones are closely linked to the nervous system. Premenstrual syndrome (PMS) can take many forms, from water retention and abdominal cramps to pounding headaches and lower back pain. It can trigger migraines and affect reasoning power. My personal view is that a lot of women have problems with their menstrual cycles because they continue to work and exercise at full pelt just before and during their periods, although nature has asked them to slow down. Some women find that PMS is much less noticeable on holiday, which is an indication that, for them, relaxation and an avoidance of pressure could alleviate the symptoms at other times.

Before a period the swollen uterus presses on major blood vessels, slowing down circulation (as in pregnant women who have swelling in the legs). Sluggish circulation leads to swollen veins and a depot of blood in the pelvic region. This deprives the brain of blood (just as a heavy meal does), and if blood flow to the brain is further restricted by vertebral artery compression, the brain feels agitated, which is the root cause of premenstrual syndrome.

Dietary guidance

Heavy demands on your digestive system will drain your energy and divert blood – and therefore oxygen – from your brain. So it makes sense to eat lighter foods in the days leading up to the start of your period. **Before your period:**
• Eat plenty of vegetables and fish or, temporarily, a vegetarian diet.
• Have juices and fruit to provide glucose (see illustration opposite).
• Avoid alcohol, coffee and energy drinks, which are often high in caffeine.
Once your period has started:
• Take special care to drink plenty of water, herbal teas etc.; don't try to cut down because you are feeling bloated from water retention.
• Balance your low-protein intake of the past few days with plenty of easily digestible protein. Chicken soup made with stock from the chicken carcass is especially good (see page 153).
• Avoid fatty foods and highly spiced foods that will stay in your system for a long time.
• Continue to abstain from caffeine, and also salty foods and those high in citric acid.
• Avoid cold foods, especially ice cream and cold water, as the chill can cause spasms in the uterus.

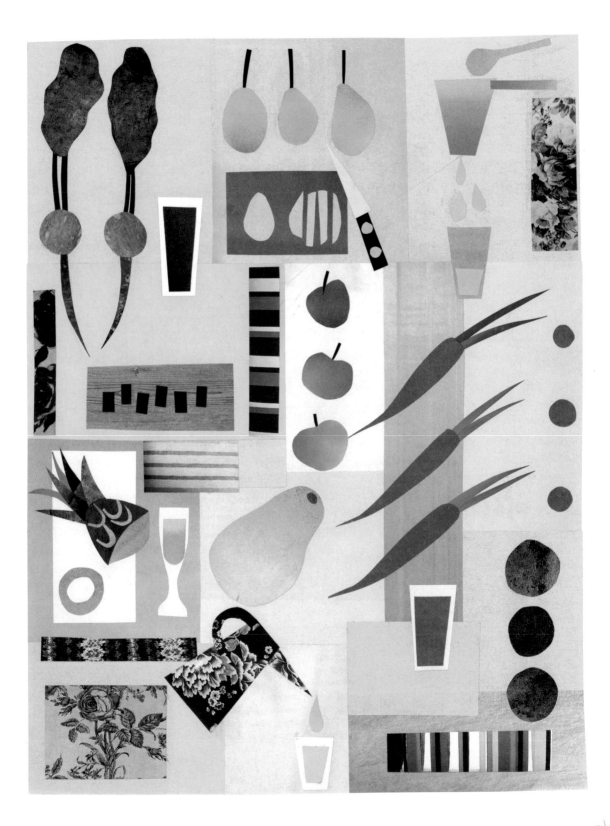

For two weeks after your period:
This is when the endometrium, the lining of the womb, is building up, so your diet should be perfectly balanced.
• Include pomegranate, carrot juice, calves' liver and protein in your diet.
• Other good ingredients include spinach and red apples for iron, and yams for phytoestrogen.
• This is the ideal time to take supplements. Some women take a lot of vitamin B complex and E supplements for premenstrual tension, but that's the wrong time. The right time is during and after the periods, when the body really needs them.

Weight-reducing diets never take account of the hormonal cycle. This sort of thing should only be done around and after the midcycle, i.e. not more than fourteen days per month. Fasting should also be avoided around the menstrual period.

the menopause

The time during which the body adjusts to new hormonal balances with the onset of the menopause brings a variety of symptoms, of which erratic and then absent menstruation is only one. Hot flushes, especially at night, uncontrollable mood swings, headaches and a dry vagina are other common and unpleasant effects of this period of change. As with PMS, the experience is not the same for everyone.

Follow a largely vegetarian diet and only have proteins in the form of fish and meat once or twice a week (also see PMS pages 186–8).

Other beneficial treatments

• Women who have neck and shoulder massages before their periods feel a lot better and more relaxed.

INFERTILITY

Of course, infertility is not going to be cured at a stroke by a simple change in diet, but diet-related conditions such as iron deficiency or being underweight can adversely affect an ability to conceive. And since what you eat and drink fashions the environment inside your body it makes sense to ensure that this environment is as receptive to sperm and to a newly created embryo as possible.

Dietary guidance

I believe that acidic and spicy food may change the pH level of the vaginal area, and if it becomes too acidic it will act like a spermicide. Avoid:
• Acidic fruits such as citrus fruits, pineapple, excess raspberries or strawberries.
• Tomato juice.
• Vinegar.
• Excess garlic.
• Highly spiced dishes.
• Canned food and drinks and ready-prepared

products, which often contain citric acid or other acidic preservatives.
• White wine, champagne, brandy, spirits etc.

Some foods and drinks produce large amounts of abdominal gas, which may disturb pelvic circulation. For this reason, it is sensible to cut out:
• Fizzy drinks, including beer and champagne.
• Yeast products.
• Sugary food and drinks.

Stress can be an effective barrier to conception. Cut down on coffee, and to help you relax follow the Regimen Therapy (see chapter 7), which incorporates several measures to relieve stress. Also see Other beneficial treatments on page 189.

Ensure your diet includes sufficient protein. The synthesis of blood and hormones, the development of egg cells in the ovaries, and the growth of the inner lining of the womb all involve proteins and cannot be wholly replaced by other foodstuffs. Animal proteins are preferable, and oestrogen is synthesised from a cholesterol-based product found only in animal fat protein.

Vitamin E is fat-soluble and is present in abundance in egg and animal protein.

Make sure you are getting plenty of vitamins and minerals in your diet, especially iron and cobalt. These help blood synthesis, vital for women of reproductive age.

Helpful nutritional supplements

• Mexican yam capsules are helpful in regulating long cycles, over 35 days. (A cycle of between 24 and 30 days, with a flow lasting for four to five days is considered normal and Mexican yam should not be taken.) I personally believe that a fertile woman, provided her partner's sperm count and quality are not a problem, should focus on the length of the cycle and duration of the menstrual period. Mexican yam is the herbal alternative to progesterone, which prepares the endometrium (the lining of the womb) to receive a fertilised egg.

• For an effective Indian herbal remedy, mix 1 tsp shatavari powder (or 2 tablets on their own), ¼ tsp kolonji oil, 7–8 saffron stamens and 1 tsp honey; take with warm milk after breakfast.

• Shatavari is a traditional Indian herb containing phytoestrogen, which mimics the functions of oestrogen. It helps to regulate periods and improve the lining of the womb. Used for centuries, this herb, along with aloe vera, is a favourite prescription for women's problems.

• Kolonji oil (*Nigella sativa*) is a traditional multi-purpose tonic that boosts the body's energy levels. The Prophet Mohammed mentioned the seeds and the oil in the Hadidth, a collection of advice on the art of living. In the Arab world, kolonji oil is traditionally used by women to improve the quality of their periods, but it has numerous other uses.

• Saffron is another energy booster. It is a powerful 'heating' herb, and helps to improve periods, libido, digestion and energy. A weak woman with anaemia, low blood pressure, poor appetite and extremely low energy levels finds it difficult to conceive.

Other beneficial treatments

Stress is a foremost indirect cause of infertility. Tenseness can cause physical constrictions all over the body, including the neck (affecting blood flow to the pituitary gland, which stimulates ovulation), the fallopian tubes and the uterus. Homeopathy, acupuncture, yoga and meditation are all good stress relievers.

Over-vigorous and muscle-building exercises can interfere with fertility. Instead, exercise such as pilates, walking, swimming and dancing are invigorating yet calming.

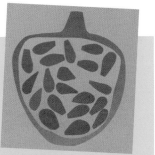

pomegranates

This fruit was traditionally recommended by certain Indian herbalists for treating infertility. If you look closely at a pomegranate seed you will see that it resembles the shape of a womb, with a small spherical bulb in the centre representing the foetus. This, they reasoned, was nature's hint that the fruit was good for women who were either pregnant or trying to conceive. What we now know is that pomegranates contain high levels of iron and especially cobalt, which contributes to its colour. Cobalt is an essential raw material for the synthesis of blood, and an important factor for pregnant women. The endometrium or womb lining, where the actual implant of a fertilised egg takes place, almost entirely consists of blood.

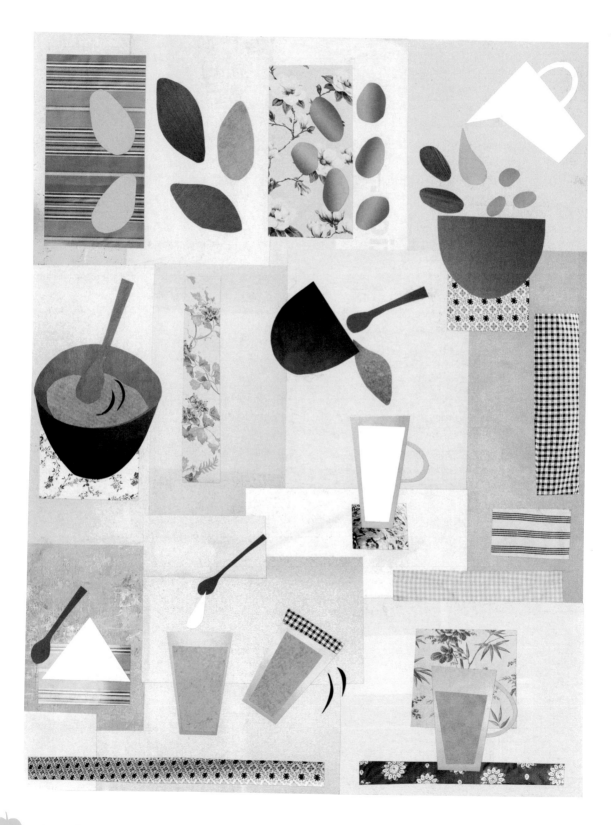

MALE INFERTILITY

Like female infertility, erectile problems or a low sperm count (the two are not necessarily synonymous) can stem from a variety of causes or combinations of causes, many of them outside the realm of nutrition. Check with your physician that the pituitary functions, testosterone level, sperm count and sperm quality are unaffected. If these tests do not reveal any problems, try the following measures:
• Follow the Regimen Therapy (see chapter 7) for a nutritionally rich diet and use regular relaxation techniques (stress is a barrier to successful sex).
• Ensure your diet isn't deficient in vitamins A, B, C or E, or minerals selenium and zinc (see pages 16–21).
• Increase the protein from meat, fish and eggs in your diet. Egg increases sperm production: follow a very lightly boiled egg with a glass of full-fat milk.

• Add saffron to hot milk or puddings.
• Take a spoonful of dry ginger powder mixed with honey at bedtime.
• Thandai is a highly potent drink traditionally used by men in India to improve their overall sex power. To make it (see illustration opposite), soak almonds and pistachios for 24 hours and grind to a paste. Stir into a glass of cold milk, add sugar and shake well or combine in a blender (the grinding and shaking potentiates the nuts and increases their effectiveness).
• The best time to make love is very early in the morning, when you are relaxed and your senses and erogenous zones are at their most sensitive.
    See also page 101 for information on xeno-oestrogens.

VAGINAL THRUSH

The itchy sensation and thick white discharge of vaginal thrush (candidiasis) is caused by a yeast infection, which erupts when the balance of 'good' bacteria and yeast in the body is upset. Such an imbalance is caused by killing off the bacteria, which can happen if we take antibiotics, or by 'overdosing' on yeast products. It is more likely to strike when we are run-down or ill.

Dietary guidance

Avoid all yeast, fungal foods and sugars. These include:
• Bread and pizza.
• Blue cheeses and soft cheeses with rinds.
• Grapes and dried fruit.
• Yeast extracts.
• Sugary foods.
• Alcohol, especially beer.
• Mushrooms.
    Follow the dietary guidelines in the Regimen Therapy (chapter 7) to make sure you are getting

the most from your food, as a healthy body can fight off infections like thrush more effectively.
• Combine protein with vegetables and restrict carbohydrates to a minimum.
• Eat live yoghurt regularly to help build up 'friendly' bacteria.

Helpful nutritional supplements

• Kadu (*Helleborus niger*). Soak 2–3 twigs in a cup of hot water and leave overnight. Strain and drink in the morning. Repeat daily for 2–3 months.
• Capsules of caprylic acid or grape seed oil (consult your physician).
• Infusions of vitamin C and B$_{12}$ intravenously helps to boost the body.
• Acidophyllus with bifidus capsules.

Other helpful treatments

Soak a wad of cotton wool in live yoghurt and insert it into the vagina; leave for a few hours.

chapter 22
immunological health

Everything that enters the body is foreign to it: food, drinks, fungal spores, germs, pollen, dust, medicines, chemicals, gases, even cosmetics. The immune system is there to deal with these 'invasions' every moment of our lives. Normally it does its job silently and without our noticing, but if it becomes overloaded (as can happen during the hay fever season) or there is some collateral disease, the immune system becomes highly sensitised.

At this stage, the slightest hint from an allergic substance in the food or air will result in a massive over-reaction from the body to eliminate it. This allergic reaction may take the form of increased mucus secretion, constriction of the bronchial tract or skin eruptions. Sometimes the reaction is so severe that it can stop the heart. This is called anaphylactic shock and super-sensitised people carry adrenaline or steroid injections to block this potentially fatal reaction of the immune system.

Sometimes it is not a foreign body that brings the immune system out fighting, but the body's own tissues. If an infection or a chemical substance changes the nature of proteins in the cells of a tissue to the extent that they are not recognised as the body's own, the immune system will develop antibodies to attack these defective cells or tissues. This turning of the body on itself is called auto-immune disease and it can affect many different parts of the body, from the salivary and tear glands (Syogren's disease) or the thyroid (Hashimoto's disease) to internal organs (systemic lupus) and the joints (rheumatoid arthritis, described on page 171. Covered here are Crohn's disease and ulcerative colitis, auto-immune diseases that affect the bowels.

ASTHMA

In sensitised people, an asthmatic attack may be started by dust mites, pet hair, pollen, certain foods or a whole host of irritants. The body reacts by releasing a flood of mucus and constricting the respiratory passages. The result might vary from gentle wheezing and a slightly tight feeling in the chest to an acute seizure that makes breathing almost impossible.

Asthma often goes hand in hand with eczema (see page 197) and even plays 'hide and seek' in the same person, with the breathing regulating itself for a while and the dry, itchy skin of eczema flaring up instead.

Asthma is most common in children, and becoming more so. Children with poor immune systems who have been exposed to a lot of antibiotics or who were not breastfed beyond a month have a tendency towards asthma and/or eczema. There seems to be a genetic predisposition towards the condition, and I have also observed amazingly close links between birth experience and immunological problems. From questioning parents over the past 15 years I have established that children with asthma or eczema frequently have a history of mild cranial-neck damage at birth through forceps or ventouse delivery, a rapid 'champagne cork' birth (under two hours) or an extremely slow birth (over 20 hours).

Perhaps in such births the pituitary and hypothalamus, controlling the immune system, receive less cerebro-spinal fluid and blood supply along the vertebral arteries.

It has been observed that children with the worst allergies come from the cleanest homes, so there is a need to strike a balance between protection from germs and disease and exposure to the realities of the environment to develop a healthy immune system.

The guidance below is particularly aimed at children, and they respond well, as do people who have developed asthma as adults (but usually before the age of forty). Many children 'grow out' of asthma but some never do. Adults who are lifelong sufferers respond least well to treatment, but following the guidelines below together with Regimen Therapy (see chapter 7), conventional medication and, especially, yoga breathing exercises offers the best combination of treatment for asthma.

Dietary guidance

Asthma sufferers can use diet in two ways: to discover whether a food allergy is involved, and to avoid foods that cause conditions that will make an attack worse or more painful.

Avoid foods that increase mucus production. These include:
• Yeast in bread and dough products such as pizza, and yeast-extract spreads.
• Fungal foods such as mushrooms.
• Dairy foods (including ice cream).
• Chilled drinks.

Very cold food and drinks tend to cause more mucus production in the throat and can throw blood vessels in the tonsils and throat into spasm, making them more vulnerable to infection. Americans, in particular, are always amazed to hear that ice cubes and their favourite ice cream can encourage colds and coughs.

Avoid acid foods that irritate the throat (see Chapter 4): These include:

relieving pressure on the diaphragm

While treating hundreds of adult patients with asthma, I made a remarkable observation: most suffered from excess abdominal gas or flatulence. Such asthma patients also have slightly compressed lungs. Gas trapped in the colon pushes up the dome of the diaphragm, not only causing difficulty in breathing but also reducing the volume of the lungs. Moreover, sufferers depend heavily on the diaphragm to expel the air out of the lungs, but such a movement is hindered because the diaphragm is already raised.

Reducing the production of abdominal gases by following the Regimen Therapy (see chapter 7), in particular avoiding yeast and sugar (which feeds yeasts in the gut), allows the diaphragm to drop to its normal position and to aid exhalation. This explains why patients who forget to do their breathing exercises improve in their asthmatic condition just by following the diet.

• Fizzy juice drinks and bottled juices.
• Canned food.
• Pickled and vinegary food.
• Nuts.
• Chillies and strong spices.
• Very fatty or oily food.

Fat and oil leave a coating on the throat that makes it more susceptible to irritation and inflammation. Both the Chinese and Indians favour drinking hot tea after a fatty meal as a counter-measure – warm water 'washes' the fat or oil off the lining of the gullet and stomach, so that the body doesn't have to produce extra acid to do the job.

Avoid substances that are a common cause of intolerances or allergies (see pages 197–8). Take a test for food allergies (the test known as ELISA is one of the most reliable). Even if this does not

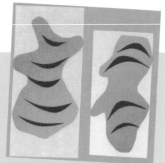

ginger

Among ginger's many powerful medicinal properties are that it aids digestion, reduces pain and fever, energises the body, and acts as an expectorant. It improves circulation, which makes it a help in overcoming nausea and dizziness (by improving cerebral circulation) and the spasms of intestinal and menstrual cramps. It is also an anti-inflammatory: dry ginger powder is used in India for arthritis and sprains or injuries. An enzyme in ginger called zingibain helps to digest protein, which makes it good for tenderising meat.

show you to be allergic to one of the foods listed, it is wise to steer clear of them. Allergies are complex in the way they work and there will quite often be no adverse reaction until a threshold is crossed.

Eat the following:
• Foods that help boost the immune system and general health as these will all help the body cope better with attacks and raise the threshold before one occurs.
• Ginger is a useful anti-allergenic and also helps to dry up mucus. The best way to use ginger is to process the root through a juicer. This juice can then be stored in the fridge and a teaspoonful mixed with a teaspoonful of organic honey and taken once or twice a day. Honey, too, has some anti-allergic properties. Root ginger is quite widely available, but if you cannot find any, powdered ginger can be used with honey in the same proportions; the juice, however, is more potent than the powder.

Feeding children

A healthy, varied and nutritious diet makes sense for all children, regardless of whether they have asthma or not. Ensuring that they get all the goodness they need while following the restrictions outlined above may require a little more thought and effort, but the time spent preparing good, home-cooked food will almost certainly mean less time spent in doctors' surgeries and it will also reduce the worry and sleeplessness of night-time attacks.

For breakfast, make various combinations of the following:
• Cereal with soya or goat's milk.
• Porridge.
• Cottage cheese.
• Soda bread, rice cakes or crispbreads.
• Pancakes.
• Honey.
• Fresh juice (not citrus).
A cup of freshly squeezed carrot and apple juice two or three times a week is a good source of vitamins and minerals. Add a little juiced ginger if they like it.

Lunch and dinner should include meat or fish, fresh vegetables and pasta, rice or potatoes (or a yeast-free bread). Children following the allergy diet will not be getting protein from dairy products, and some children are also allergic to eggs, so it is particularly important that they get plenty of protein from other sources. Protein is essential for growth, and asthmatic children are inclined to be short for their age (the pituitary gland secretes growth hormones as well as the adrenals that control the immune system, a further indicator that the pituitary gland plays a major role in controlling allergies). The steroids in their medication (see page 196) and the diversion of so much energy into breathing also affect growth. A child under ten will need 100 g of red meat, chicken or its equivalent every day, and a child over ten requires 150 g to provide a high-protein intake. Ensure the meat is lean.

For more ideas on good food for children, including alternatives to junk food and coping with food fads, see Chapters 8 and 9.

protein-packed meals for kids

Salsa bolognese   Mince chicken or turkey meat at home and make it into a fresh pasta sauce with tomatoes, onions, garlic and herbs. Make up a batch and freeze it in individual portions. As well as a sauce for spaghetti, tagliatelle or any other pasta shape, use it to stuff cannelloni or layer it with pasta sheets and shredded spinach to make lasagne. It also makes a good topping for baked potatoes.

Lamb patties   Mince lean lamb and season it with garlic, ginger, black pepper and a little salt. Bind together with a little beaten egg and press it around kebab sticks, make it into meatballs or mould it into whatever shape you like, from burgers to gingerbread men, then grill. Alternatively, you could make it into shepherd's pie by omitting the egg, adding some cooked onions and grated carrot and putting it under a blanket of mashed potato. These have all proved popular with my children and their friends when I prepare them.

Frijoles   Soak red kidney beans overnight, rinse well and boil the beans in fresh water for 30–45 minutes or until soft. Fry chopped onions, garlic and ginger in a little olive oil. Add salt to taste, then add the kidney beans and some chopped tomatoes. Continue to cook, stirring regularly, until the tomatoes have cooked down into a rich sauce. Sprinkle in some parsley. The dish makes another good topping for potatoes, or you can serve it with rice the Mexican way.

Conventional medicine

The most common treatment for asthma is to give antibiotics to kill off bacteria that have taken hold in the excess mucus in the chest (a persistent cough and one cold after another is often a sign of a tendency to asthma), followed by nebulisers or inhalers. These do alleviate the symptoms, which is necessary, but do not hit at the root cause, as most doctors will admit. Antibiotics also act as immuno-suppressants.

Many asthma preparations contain steroids in some form or another and, although it is better to stay clear of steroids, it is not advisable to stop them without medical supervision; this can even be dangerous. Explain to your doctor about the regime you are following and work with her or him to reduce the dose steadily once you are seeing positive results. Some doctors have an 'if the medicines work, don't stop them' attitude, but more are increasingly receptive to alternative treatments. A peak flow test that shows improvement in lung capacity will encourage your doctor to support you.

Helpful nutritional supplements

• Chinese herbal medicine has proved very effective with many life-long adult sufferers.
• Another successful treatment for adults is Dr Ali's Winter Tea with liquorice and other herbal supplements (see page 220). This is an Ayurvedic preparation that should be drunk as a tea twice a day for a month. This infusion is not as powerful as prescribed asthma medication, but it shows a therapeutic effect over time, increasing expectoration and dilating the bronchial tubes.

Other beneficial treatments

• Yoga, in particular breathing techniques (*pranayama*) for cleansing breath and breath retention.
• Massage of the shoulder and neck area. This relaxes the tenseness caused by the effort of breathing, and improves the circulation of cerebro-spinal fluids and the flow of blood to the pituitary gland in the base of the brain that controls the immune system.
• Acupuncture.
• Homeopathy.

Time spent preparing good, home-cooked food will almost certainly mean less time spent in doctors' surgeries.

managing your hay fever

The sneezing, runny nose and itchy eyes and throat that for many people signal the arrival of summer are not triggered specifically by hay. Sometimes a particular plant or seasonal pollutant is to blame, but often it is just that for most of the year the sensitivity is kept below a threshold you can cope with, but flares up when the combined rise of pollen, dust, sunshine and other triggers collectively form, in the body's terms, a threat. Because this is just another manifestation of an allergic reaction, all the guidelines for asthma (see pages 192–4) are helpful in reducing susceptibility to hay fever too.

Before the hay fever season starts, prepare by fasting or semi-fasting once a week with water and vegetable soup (see Chapter 6), to give the body a chance to avoid all food-related allergens that day. Totally avoid any foodstuffs or other products (perhaps certain cosmetics or smells like wet paint) that you react slightly to, as they will contribute to tipping you over the allergy threshold when the pollen count rises.

The hot, itchy skin rash of eczema can flare up in times of stress, but is most often an allergic reaction. Its links with asthma (the skin and lungs stem from the ectoderm in an embryo, which gives them shared properties) mean that one can be an alternative manifestation of the other; in some people they turn and turn about, one taking the upper hand as the other goes into abeyance.

Eczema is usually worst where there is friction – in folds of skin like the eyelids, elbows and behind the knees, between the fingers and in the groin. Children's cheeks and anal region are also commonly affected. A feature of eczema is that it will mirror itself, appearing on the left and right sides of the body in identical places.

Dietary guidance

Follow the advice given for asthma (see pages 192–4). If eczema is aggravated by stress, also avoid coffee and excess alcohol as these increase tenseness.

Other helpful treatments

• Skin creams and treatment for acne (see page 181).
• Homeopathic remedies.

Asthma often goes hand in hand with eczema.

Contact dermatitis and hives (urticaria)

These are both caused by allergic reactions. As its name implies, contact dermatitis is a rash or irritation at the point of contact with something to which you have a sensitivity. A particular brand of cosmetics or washing detergent (or a perfumed ingredient in them) and the sap from certain plants are common sources.

Hives are raised red lumps that occur when the fluid containing allergens leaks out of smaller blood vessels under the skin. It is a different manifestation of hay fever or a food allergy and should be treated in the same way. The skin-calming creams recommended for acne and eczema are helpful in relieving the swelling and itching.

FOOD INTOLERANCES AND ALLERGIES

An intolerance to a food is not the same as an allergy. An intolerance is usually related to an inability to process a food in some way, rather than the triggering of an exaggerated response from the immune system. However, if you flood your system with a food it can't cope with, crossing the tolerance threshold, this can cause sensitisation and an allergic reaction.

An intolerance to a food can manifest itself in many different ways: as abdominal bloating, diarrhoea, headaches and migraine, skin rashes, mouth ulcers or fever. The reaction can be mild (itchiness of the palate from eating pineapple) to immobilising (severe diarrhoea within 15 minutes of eating blue cheese), specific (an inability to digest milk due to a lack of the necessary enzyme) or more general (difficulty in digesting fatty food, which sits in the stomach for hours causing belching or heartburn). Some people can go in and out of intolerances.

Food intolerances are getting worse. My belief is that genetically modified foods are acting as

The obvious solution is to avoid foods to which you know you have an intolerance.

foods that 'disagree'

Here are some of the most common ingredients to which people have an intolerance:
• Dairy produce (lactose intolerance).
• Wheat (gluten intolerance; see coeliac disease, right).
• Yeast.
• Mushrooms.
• Chocolate.
• Eggs.
• Shellfish.
• Chemical additives.
• Citric acid.
• Coffee.
• Cheese.
• Pineapple.
• Chillies.
• Garlic.
• Nuts.
• Monosodium glutamate (MSG), used in commercially prepared Chinese food.
• Vinegar.
• Alcohol (particularly white wine).
• Sugary food. Sugar in general is not good for anyone when consumed in excess, but especially for someone vulnerable to food sensitivity. Sugar feeds the yeast and fungi that thrive in the gut, producing alcohols and other toxins that can sensitise the body. For some people, alcohol itself can in certain forms cause an allergic asthmatic reaction. See also Chapter 4.

'foreign bodies' in the gut. As multi-culturalism expands, people are also exposing their digestive systems to many different foods alien to the culture that shaped their constitution.

Food allergies are also increasingly problematic and often more severe in reaction than an intolerance. Nut allergies have been well-publicised and in some cases even a minute amount can set off a massive and dangerous reaction. A lot of people are badly allergic to shellfish, which highlights the problem of pollutants triggering allergic reactions. Shellfish and crustaceans thriving on the shores of major cities swallow garbage, toxic waste, heavy metals, sewage etc., which is then stored in their bodies. These are, of course, potentially very harmful.

The obvious solution is to avoid foods to which you know you have an intolerance. If you suspect an intolerance but are unsure of its source, you can be tested (see page 193). You can also experiment at home by excluding various suspects from your diet and noting any changes.

Homeopathy is also helpful in dealing with adverse reactions to food.

Coeliac disease (gluten intolerance)

One of the most common food intolerances is to gluten, a protein in wheat and rye and, to a much lesser extent, other grains. In susceptible people, gluten causes damage to the lining of the intestines, which becomes inflamed and unable to take up the nutrients it should. As well as discomfort from diarrhoea and bloating, therefore, it can result in deficiency problems such as osteoporosis, anaemia, poor vitamin absorption and, in children, poor growth.

If you suffer from a gluten intolerance, you should obviously avoid all wheat products. In addition, I have found that cutting out the following can be beneficial:
• Milk.
• Yoghurt.
• Cheese.
• Bitter beer.

To recover from an inflammation, follow the regime for diarrhoea (see pages 145–7 and 153).

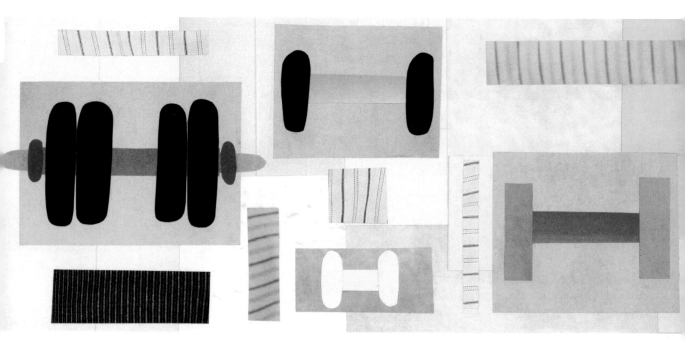

CROHN'S DISEASE AND ULCERATIVE COLITIS

These are two common auto-immune diseases that result in inflammation of the lining of the bowels. Ulcerative colitis involves the formation of ulcers on the surface of the colon, which bleed and are often painful. As the red, swollen bowels become non-functional, there is constant secretion of mucus, and stools (full of digestive juices and water) cannot firm up. Sometimes, in ulcerative colitis, there are no folds in the lining of the bowels to increase the surface area, which impairs the absorption ability of the colon. Instead, the colon's 'lead-pipe' appearance lets faecal masses go right through. Malabsorption of nutrients leads to such problems as weight loss, vitamin and mineral deficiency and anaemia.

Dietary guidance

Follow the anti-diarrhoea diet (see page 153) for 4–6 months, to help to form stools.

Helpful nutritional supplements

• Take herbal anti-diarrhoea (pech-unani) supplements twice a week for a month to slow down the motility of bowels and enable better absorption of nutrients.

Other beneficial treatments

• Vigorous muscle-building exercise – such as lifting weights (see illustration above) or jogging – encourages the gut to absorb nutrients more efficiently. In addition, it stimulates the adrenal glands to secrete excess anabolic steroids (to give more bulk to the muscles); these tissue-building steroids help to heal ulcers and inflamed bowel tissues.
• Massage of the neck and spine improves blood flow to the pituitary gland. This gland instructs the adrenal glands and the immune system to control the aggressiveness of the auto-immune reaction.

chapter 23
general health

It will be apparent by now that although some disorders have a simple, directly attributable cause, many more are multifactorial – they are brought about by a combination of factors. And our ability to heal from even something as directly attributable as a broken bone or an infectious disease will be influenced by our age, diet and general state of health.

In both succumbing to and recovering from any form of illness, energy is almost always a factor. Energy is necessary for every single function in the body. Like pain, temperature and diarrhoea, fatigue indicates the failure of a vital system. A lack of energy triggers a whole series of malfunctions, from a weakening of the immune, hormonal, circulatory and digestive systems to depression, panic attacks, memory loss and blackouts. If your energy is constantly in short supply, your body will not have the defences to fight off long-term pathogenic invasion, such as cancer. Energy, as explained in Chapter 1, comes from what we eat and drink, so the quality of our food affects our energy levels,

and our efficiency at processing it into a usable form depends on our digestive systems doing their jobs properly.

This chapter looks at conditions and syndromes that cross the boundaries and affect our entire bodies. Some, such as insomnia and the mundane headache, are not illnesses in themselves but a symptom that might have its roots in a multiplicity of problems major or minor. Others, such as cancer and chronic fatigue syndrome, are truly multifactorial. All are most responsive to a combination of several different forms of therapy. That is what integrated medicine does best.

MIGRAINE

This is more than a severe headache. It is a collection of symptoms which, as well as a blinding, one-sided headache, typically includes sensitivity to light and sounds, interference with vision, dizziness, palpitations, hyperventilation, a tender scalp and occasionally fainting and confusion. During an attack, the arteries that feed the membrane around the brain go into spasm, inhibiting blood flow and building up intercranial pressure. Vomiting is the body's way of reducing the fluid pressure in the cranium, which eases the headache, so nausea and vomiting are common. Some people find they get a warning of an attack in the form of flashing lights or a sense of anxiety; this is called migraine with aura.

The actual cause of migraine is not known, but hormonal changes (some women get migraine around their periods that then stop with the menopause), compression of the vertebral arteries and stress can all bring on an attack. Certain foods are also triggers. Some people have an attack when stress or an excess of a food or drink suddenly stops – 'withdrawal migraines' can strike on the first day of a holiday, for instance. Many migraines are cyclical in nature, occurring regularly once a week, a month and so on.

Finding the cycle or trigger for your migraine is enormously helpful – it means you can take preventative measures that will at first make the attacks less severe and then less frequent. An attack itself can be quite debilitating, so all efforts should be made to relieve the symptoms, including conventional medicine. Regimen Therapy (see chapter 7), combined with osteopathy, acupuncture or homeopathy and drugs to ease the acute headaches, seems to be the best way of controlling attacks.

Some of the new drugs available are very efficient in controlling migraines. Although they are expensive, they work quite quickly. Most thin the blood so that during an attack, when the arteries are in spasm, it can flow more easily to the brain membrane. A migraine is an acute condition and, in the case of cluster migraines in particular, conventional medical treatment can bring fast relief when used alongside the other approaches described below. Sometimes oxygen is used to relieve severe headaches, indicating that a deficiency of oxygen is the cause.

Dietary guidance

If you suspect a food may be a trigger for attacks, experiment by excluding various possibilities one at a time: the usual suspects are cheese, chocolate, alcohol and caffeine.

About three days before an anticipated attack go on a one-day fruit and vegetables fast (see page 57). It is best not to do a complete water-only fast as the toxins released may trigger an attack and fasting can bring on a headache.

For the next two days avoid:
• Coffee.
• Sugar.
• Cheese and milk.
• Yeast products.
• Shellfish.
• Citrus fruits.
• Canned or preserved products.
• Fried food.
• Spicy food.
• Nuts.
• MSG.
• Alcohol.

cluster migraines

Some people find that, for a certain period, they will get attacks at a fixed time – perhaps 11 am every day for a week, and then nothing for several months or a year. This onslaught is fairly difficult to control once it has started, so take advantage of the predictable nature of the attacks well in advance, rather than waiting for the first attack.

For four to six weeks before the expected attacks, do a one-day water-only fast once a week. Then, for at least a month before the onset, adhere strictly to Regimen Therapy (see chapter 7).

During an attack eat very simply. The stomach is often upset from vomiting and needs easily digested foods such as:
• Vegetable soups.
• Porridge made with water.
• Soft-boiled eggs.
• Mashed potatoes and puréed vegetables.
• Grilled fish.
• Bananas.
• Apples and pears.

In particular, avoid acidic and spicy foods, as greater acidity in the stomach may increase the tendency to vomit.

Drink plenty of water, but sip it to avoid nausea, and drink chamomile and peppermint tea.

Helpful nutritional supplements

• 10 drops of valerian twice a day for three days from the onset of the first symptoms.

Other beneficial treatments

Follow this regime during the three-day period before an anticipated attack:
• Have at least one deep tissue massage of the neck and shoulders to improve blood flow to the head. This also helps relax the neck,

Few people can claim never to have had a headache, even a brief one. Like all forms of pain a headache is a signal or warning that something is wrong. The location of the pain can be helpful in tracking down the cause. For example:

Source of pain	Causes may include
Forehead	Tension or stress; sinus problems; weak eyesight; photosensitivity; susceptibility to radiation (from x-rays, electronic gadgets etc.).
One side of head	Migraine; whiplash; toothache; tightening of or injury to the biting muscles or jaw; constriction of vertebral artery; inflammation of the jaw joint.
Back of the skull	Injury, tension or inflammation of neck muscles; high blood pressure uncontrolled by medicine; dislocation of joints of the cervical spine; twisted neck due to sleeping badly or poor posture (particularly sitting at a computer); neuralgia of occipital nerve.
Top of the skull all over	High or low blood pressure (varies according to the intensity); anaemia; increased pressure of the brain fluid; allergy or reaction to something like wet paint; low or high blood sugar; dehydration; altitude sickness; insomnia; chronic fatigue; hangover.

A headache is also one of the symptoms of serious conditions such as brain aneurisms, meningitis and brain tumours, but statistically it is much more likely to be caused by stress, blocked sinuses, eyestrain, sudden exertion (which might be physical labour, a bout of coughing, sexual excitement or just a sudden movement), some sort of strain or a misalignment in the neck ('exertion headaches' are a common sign of this). Food-affected headaches include those brought about by:
• Internal pressure caused by constipation (see pages 140–41), high blood pressure (see pages 172–5) or sinusitis (see page 164).
• Low blood sugar (see page 176).

• Allergies and food intolerances (see pages 197–8).
   Particularly helpful in relieving headaches are:
• Neck and shoulder massage.
• Manipulative techniques such as osteopathy (especially cranial osteopathy) or chiropractic.
• Acupuncture.
• Homeopathy (spigella, staphysagria and belladonna in various potencies).
• Ginger and chamomile tea (see illustration opposite) is a great calmant and restorative.

Conventional medicines such as aspirin can relieve a headache, but try alternatives first, as the suggestions above are more likely to get to the cause of the problem.

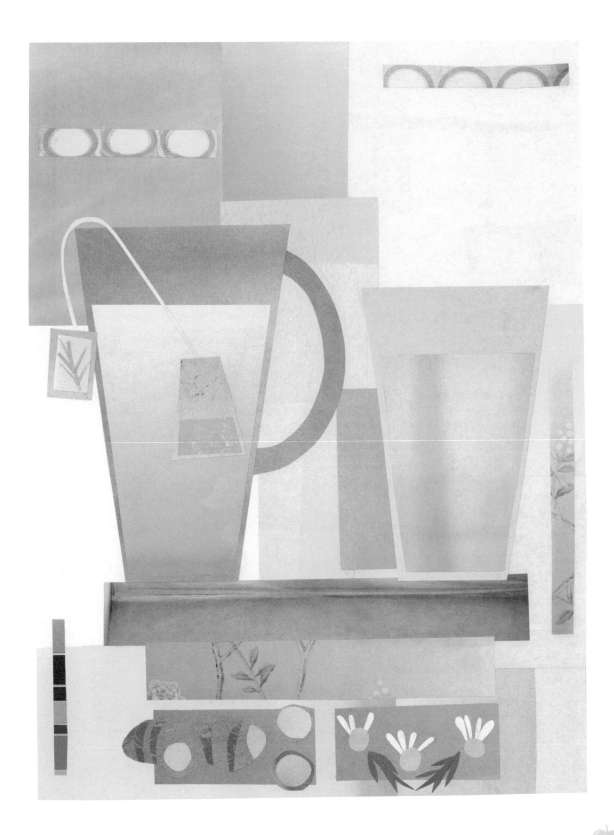

which stiffens up prior to an attack.
• Spend 10–15 minutes each morning doing yoga exercises.
• Walk or swim if you get the opportunity.
• Avoid late nights.
• Eat early (by 8 pm at the latest) and eat slowly. As far as possible avoid eating out.
• Go out of your way to avoid confrontational and stressful situations.
• A pillow in bed will improve blood circulation to the head.
• If you are regularly working at a computer, take particular care to take breaks often.
• Drink 1½–2 litres of water a day.

During an attack:
• Massage and relaxation are of utmost importance.
• Rest in bed as much as possible.
• Put a cold pack on the forehead for five minutes every two hours until the headache stops.
• Put a hot water bottle, wrapped in a towel, under the neck to release tension and improve blood flow.
• Keep the windows open to allow fresh air in.

Other beneficial treatments

The following therapies can be beneficial both before and during an attack:

chamomile

Chamomile tea is well known as a calmant or soporific. Its ability to relax muscles causes the blood pressure to drop slightly, which has a calming effect on the body. Its anti-inflammatory properties help to heal stomach ulcers and are useful in the treatment of rheumatoid arthritis and some auto-immune problems. Chamomile cream soothes burns.

• Acupuncture.
• Homeopathy.
• Head massage with Ayurvedic oils.
• Osteopathic (including cranial) and chiropractic manipulation.
• Ozone therapy.
• Oxygen (administered by a qualified professional).

SLEEP DISORDERS

Sleep is essential for everybody. Our body needs a period of complete rest in order to recover and to maintain itself. But how much sleep we require varies from person to person. Older people seem to need less, and the quality of sleep is more important than the quantity of time spent in bed.

Doctors define sleep as abnormal or insufficient when it affects day-time functioning. A lack of sleep or poor-quality sleep makes us irritable and prone to mood swings, affects our ability to concentrate and slows our reflexes.

Serious sleep deprivation can induce drunken-like behaviour and loss of balance. It is important, however, to distinguish between the tiredness caused by lack of sleep, and fatigue as a symptom of a multifactorial condition.

In addition to insomnia, sleep disorders include sleep apnoea (in which breathing unaccountably stops), restless leg syndrome, jet lag and – the opposite of insomnia – narcolepsy.

How much sleep you need depends in part on your constitution (see chapter 13) – some people are badly affected by a single disturbed night, but others seem to shrug off sleepless nights without concern. As long as you get a reasonable total, to which an afternoon siesta may be added, then there should be no problem. Just three hours sleep per night every night or many consecutive nights of broken sleep indicates something is wrong. Poor or disturbed sleep can be down to many things, from noisy neighbours (a particular problem with shiftworkers trying to sleep during the day) to lack of oxygen at high altitudes or a psychiatric disturbance such as schizophrenia. Most common, however, are:

• Working late, or getting involved in problems in the evening that fire up your brain late at night.
• Worries in your life that are difficult to put aside when you go to bed.
• An uncomfortable or unfamiliar bed.
• A bedroom that is too hot or too cold, or airless.
• A restless or snoring partner.
• Pain.
• Indigestion or disturbances from your digestion working in the middle of the night.
• Thirst.
• Certain conditions, such as chronic fatigue syndrome, that may make you tired during the day and wakeful at night.
• Too many electrical gadgets, such as a television, computer or music system, in the bedroom.

Sleep patterns are also a matter of habit, so a problem may continue even after the original cause has passed.

There is no universal remedy for sleep problems. The causes of insomnia are many, so examine your lifestyle to try to find out what may be precipitating your sleeplessness.

If insomnia is affecting you badly, consult your doctor for sleeping pills, but be warned – they are addictive. Strong sleeping pills of course overrule everything and knock you out chemically.

Dietary guidance

To promote good sleeping habits in general, follow my Regimen Therapy (see chapter 7). This will help you to avoid many of the common pitfalls that make for a disturbed night.

Certain drugs and alcohol cause sleep disorders. Caffeine is the most common cause of insomnia, as in susceptible people it causes muscles to tense up and makes relaxation difficult. Although nicotine has an initial relaxing effect, it later interferes with sleep as it irritates the brain. Alcohol similarly increases drowsiness at first, but it is very dehydrating, so someone who has fallen asleep after drinking too much will often be woken about three hours later by a raging thirst. Drugs such as cocaine and ecstasy keep the brain and body awake.

Dietary problems may not inhibit your getting off to sleep but may wake you in the middle of the night. Avoid:

• A heavy dinner, especially late at night. Unfinished digestive processes starting up again in the early hours can wake you (see pages 32–3). If indigestion or a grumbling stomach regularly wakes you even after an ordinary meal, get into the habit of a short walk after dinner, to kick-start the digestion process.
• Anything too acid or that may cause excessive flatulence (see pages 144–5) or constipation (see pages 140–44). All these conditions can lead to wakeful or disturbed nights.
• Hot sweet drinks. These are initially comforting and often recommended at bedtime, but the sugar agitates the brain rather than calming it.
• Middle-of-the-night thirst. Those who do stressful or heavy physical work during the day have a particular demand for fluids even at night. Dehydration sends the pulse racing, which is a major cause of being awoken by unnamed anxieties. Drink some water before going to bed and keep a glass of water by the bedside.

Helpful nutritional supplements

Try any of the following in consultation with a doctor or qualified herbalist and see which suits you. Be prepared to change if a solution loses its effectiveness after a while.

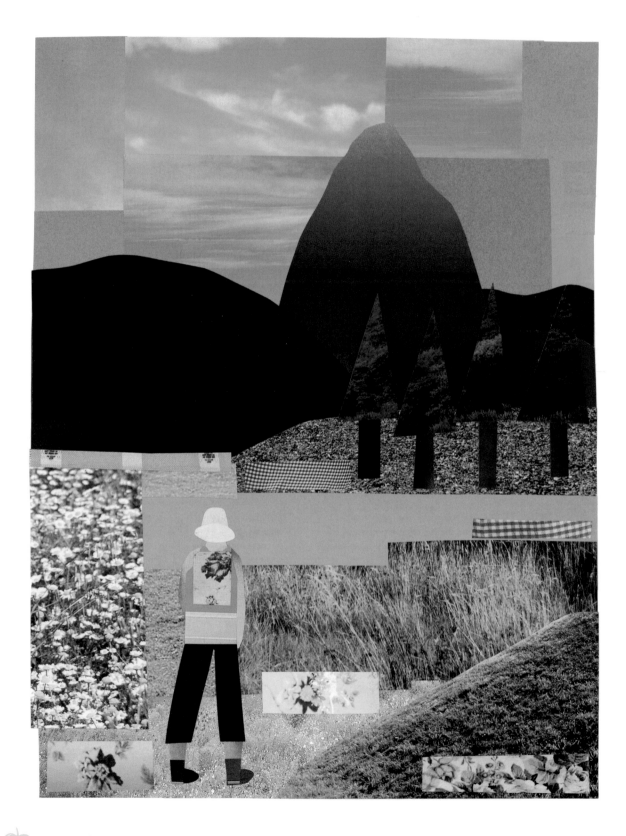

- 10–15 drops of valerian in half a cup of water at bedtime.
- 10–15 drops of Passiflora.
- 10–15 drops Avena sativa in water at bedtime.

Other beneficial treatments

- Homeopathy. Take advice from a qualified homeopath, but a combination I often recommend with success was given to me by an old Indian homeopath: take 2 tablets of Nux Vomica on the tongue at bedtime followed five minutes later by 2 tablets of Belladonna 30. You can repeat this formula if you wake up in the night and cannot get back to sleep.
- Ayurvedic medicine: 1/2 tsp each of powdered shankh puspi and jatamansi boiled in a glass of water for five minutes. Strain, cool and drink at bedtime.
- Acupuncture.
- Brahmi oil massage of the head at bedtime.

CHRONIC FATIGUE SYNDROME

A syndrome is a recognised collection of symptoms for which no single cause has been discovered. Chronic fatigue syndrome (CFS) has been given such names as 'yuppie flu' and, since many of the symptoms are psychological, has frequently been categorised as a psychiatric disorder and treated with anti-depressants. These often make patients feel better because of the 'lift' they give, but do not help the broad spectrum of CFS.

In my opinion CFS is a multifactorial condition, to which the following may contribute:

Epstein Barr virus. This triggers CFS in up to 30 per cent of cases. It is a virus that competes with the body for energy and enters mitochondria (the energy-producing 'power stations' inside cells) and destroys them. This results in every organ and system becoming sluggish – the body is nearly paralysed from within. Sufferers are barely able to move; they ache from an accumulation of lactic acid (since mitochondria are not burning glucose with oxygen) and mental activity is impaired. The presence of the virus in the tonsils and lymph glands causes frequent fever and swelling. Recovery is slow – patients can continue to suffer for years even though viral activity is negligible. This is the severest form of CFS, called myalgic encephalomyelitis (ME), which is a misnomer, because it means 'inflammation of the brain and nerve tissues causing muscle pain'. This is not the case. It is simply a serious variant of CFS.

Poor supply of glucose and oxygen to the brain. A brain struggling to function on less glucose and oxygen than it requires will result in memory loss, lack of concentration, headaches and depression as well as physical fatigue. A reduced flow of blood (which carries glucose and oxygen to the brain) has been found in about 60 per cent of CFS sufferers. The brain receives its blood supply from two sources. The carotid artery supplies the face, skull and the conscious part of the brain (cortex), controlling movement, feeling, psyche, vision, speech, hearing etc. The two vertebral arteries run one up each side of the spine, protected within a bony canal. These supply blood to the subconscious brain or brain stem and base. When these arteries are slightly compressed due to misalignment of the cervical spine – which can happen after a whiplash injury – symptoms include fatigue, headache, emotional problems, unbalance, tinnitus (ringing in the ears), panic attacks, palpitations and pituitary malfunction. As many of these symptoms are shared with CFS, I postulated that vertebral misalignment in the neck may also bring about CFS, and through neck massage, manipulation and exercises I have indeed been able to treat those symptoms in CFS sufferers.

Nutritional deficiency. Another characteristic feature of CFS is a deficiency of minerals and often vitamins. Whether this is cause or effect is not known, but I suspect that sufferers have this problem before the syndrome is manifested and it lays them open to viral complications. When suffering from CFS, the fatigue is so serious that absorption of nutrients becomes very sluggish, and vitamin and mineral therapy, especially through infusions, have helped many sufferers of CFS.

Yeast/fungal overgrowth. Some sufferers of CFS say their heads become fuzzy and they complain of severe fatigue a couple of hours after a meal. Such people are very intolerant to wine – just a sip can cause drowsiness and lethargy. Candida overgrowth in the gut inhibits absorption of nutrients and creates conditions in the gut in which toxic alcohols are produced, leading to the symptoms of deep fatigue, bloating and poor digestion of which many CFS sufferers complain. If the fungal growth penetrates the gut's lining, it allows certain toxins to enter the bloodstream, causing skin rashes, chronic fatigue and other neurological or psychological symptoms.

Other, less frequent contributors to CFS include stress, hormonal malfunction, geopathic stress (living near electronic gadgets and high-powered electric cables etc.), insomnia, IBS, chronic sinusitis and low blood pressure.

Repairing and rectifying the system is not an easy task and can take a long time. Energy levels will fluctuate, and a reasonable day may be followed by a couple of days of very poor stamina. Learn to ration your energy, or your fatigue after too much exertion (which may not, in normal terms, amount to very much effort) will be uncontrollable. This frustrating and unpredictable lassitude can be very depressing. There is no guarantee that the body will recover fully and it may be necessary to make a long-term or permanent adaptation to a slower lifestyle.

Young people recover more quickly for obvious reasons, while spinal deformation that permanently restricts blood flow to the brain (osteoporosis can do this) will hinder the chance of making a good recovery. As with all multifactorial illnesses, CFS requires treatment of the whole body, and nutrition is a vital part of successful recovery.

Dietary guidance

An essential step on the road to recovery is to give the body a boost of energy. A kick-start encourages the body's own energy-producing system to function, and Regimen Therapy (see chapter 7) can do just that. It also elicits a feel-good factor, without which a return to normal will be an uphill struggle.

Avoid anything that encourages tenseness or depression such as:
• Yeast.
• Citrus and acidic foods.
• Alcohol.
• Fried food.
• Coffee.
• Smoking.

Eat carefully structured meals:
• A good breakfast of protein, cereals and fruits.
• Lunch should also consist of protein (fish or chicken), carbohydrates (rice, pasta or potatoes) and a green salad.
• Dinner should be light as night-time sleep is essential. Something like stir-fried vegetables with rice or a bowl of pasta and some fruit as dessert.
• If finances permit, a teaspoon of caviar on a rye crispbread, rice cake or oatmeal biscuit twice a week will provide a protein and salt combination to boost the energy. Do not have this every day or it may interfere with your body's other requirements.

Drink energy-packed fluids:
• A cup of chicken soup (see page 153) an hour before the two main meals. This is an energy-giving drink full of nutrients.
• One glass a day of sweet lime juice (if available).
• Apple and pomegranate juice (or, better, eat the whole fruits).

• Ginseng or Bio Energy tea (see page 220), 1–2 cups a day as an adaptogenic beverage.
• A tablespoon of brandy in a mug of warm water, with a teaspoon of honey. Sip before dinner or half-an-hour before sleep. This will relax the muscles and induce sleep without causing any dehydration. Have this 2–3 times a week only.
• 1–2 glasses a day of whey (see page 174), to help eliminate toxins.

Helpful nutritional supplements

• Injections or suppositories of vitamins and minerals (vitamins B_{12} and C, calcium, magnesium and selenium), to boost energy. Absorption of these nutrients through the gut is likely to be poor. Once a level of improvement has been reached, these can be continued as oral supplements.

Other beneficial treatments

• Massage and manipulation of the neck.
• Acupuncture.
• I have found that walking at altitude is an almost miraculous cure for CFS (see illustration on page 206).

CANCER

The integrated medical approach to cancer is the subject of a book in itself, so what follows should be regarded as no more than guidelines.

Cancer is a multifactorial disease. Some substances are carcinogenic, that is, they cause certain body cells to mutate and multiply, impeding the body from functioning normally and killing regular cells. But the rules are not the same for everyone – we have all heard smokers who are reluctant to give up declare that they had a grandfather or an aunt who 'smoked like a chimney all his or her life yet was hale and hearty to the age of 94'. What seems clear is that (major radioactive contamination or similar uncommon accidents apart) it usually takes a combination of factors to trigger cells into mutating: genetics, stress levels, general health and diet are all major players. And the same apparent circumstances may result in different outcomes – one person under chronic stress may develop psoriasis, while another may develop cancer.

The prognosis for cancer has improved in recent years, helped by early diagnosis. Eradicating cancer is very much more difficult and uncertain once cancer cells have travelled to different parts of the body and started new colonies, known as secondaries or metastatic cancer areas. There are growing reports of cancer survivors and people who have gone into long remission. When I was practising in India I had over a hundred cancer patients who exceeded normal survival expectations, some by many years. At the Integrated Medical Centre we have dozens of cases of cancer which have gone into remission; some patients have been symptom-free for over five years, the deadline to be regarded as a cure. We work hand in hand with conventional medical doctors, liaising with them throughout the treatment wherever possible.

My approach is that when one does not know what causes an ailment it is best to look after the body and mind to maintain an equilibrium. The body's sanogenetic powers are strong and if the right conditions are laid down then the body balances by itself and restores health. Regimen Therapy (see chapter 7) offers two approaches. Used as an alternative, the remissions achieved are comparable with those obtained by conventional medicine. As a complement to chemotherapy, it achieves substantial improvements in the quality of life and probably the best overall prospects of extended remission. Willpower is an essential component of healing, but it is not enough just to say 'I'll fight it': you have to do things to aid the body's own healing power.

protect yourself from cancer

Managing your health and controlling your stress levels can go a long way to keeping the body's defences in good condition. Although there is nothing miraculous that can specifically prevent cancer, the following steps will help you to guard against it:

• Eat organic food.
• Avoid smoking.
• Avoid drinking excess alcohol and coffee.
• Follow the Regimen Therapy (see chapter 7).

What you eat and drink can also do much to alter the odds:

• Antioxidants help limit the proliferation of damaging free radicals. You can increase your supply of antioxidants by eating plenty of fresh fruit and vegetables, especially red, orange and yellow ones like peppers, carrots, beetroot and tomatoes (see illustration opposite); dark green leafy vegetables like watercress; nuts; and oily fish.

• The onion family, especially garlic and onions, may provide protection against cancers, in particular of the stomach.

• Amla is a fruit that grows wild in India, but is available through Ayurvedic outlets. In Sanskrit it is called 'sustainer of life'. Its extremely high vitamin C content means it is a powerful antioxidant. Amla can be cooked with vegetables or steeped in syrup. It is one of the main ingredients of the ancient Ayurvedic tonic known as chawanprash (see page 220) and the dried fruit are used in the Ayurvedic powder called triphala ('three fruits': amla, hirada and behera), used to treat irritable bowel syndrome and to promote general good health as well as to fortify against cancers.

• Avoid eating highly charred food (crispy barbecues, dark toast) and smoked food. Burning and smoking food changes its chemical make-up and can create carcinogenic elements not present in the food in its usual form.

• Cured and smoked meats and fish often attract all sorts of bacteria and fungal spores present in the air. As these develop, they produce toxic waste which remains on the surface of the food, which can in turn produce a toxic effect in the gut, liver and elsewhere. Smoked fish is known to cause naso-pharyngeal cancers, sometimes called 'Shanghai cancer' because it occurs more frequently in China, where people consume a lot of cured fish.

• The long-term effects of artificial additives, fertilisers, pesticides and growth enhancers have yet to be fully identified. Avoid them by eating fresh, organic produce whenever possible.

• Don't put extra stress on your body by becoming very overweight: obesity is a factor in some cancers and is never compatible with optimum health.

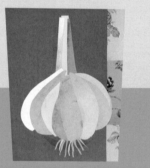

garlic

The medicinal powers of garlic are legendary, from decongesting a blocked nose to contributing to longevity. It reduces cholesterol; lowers blood pressure; strengthens the immune system; helps to stimulate bile, therefore aiding digestion; keeps candida growth in check; and is proving an effective guard against certain sorts of cancer. Allicin, which gives garlic its characteristic smell, has antibacterial and fungicidal properties. Because the smell of garlic on the breath can be offputting, a variety of deodorised garlic capsules, pills and other forms of supplements have become available, but these do not have anything like the same level of beneficial effect as the fresh bulb, which is at its most powerful when eaten raw.

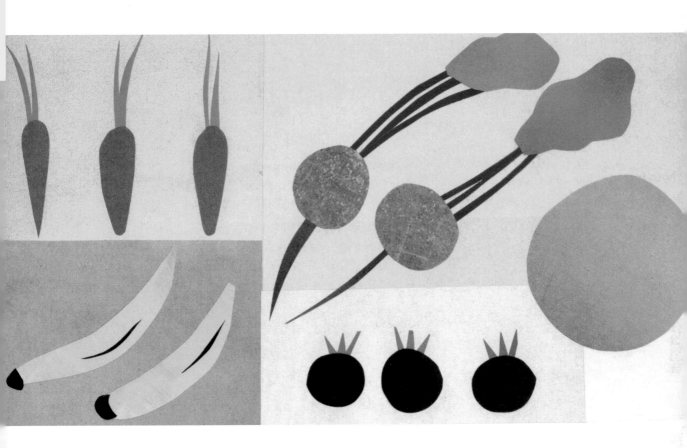

Dietary guidance

Chemotherapy puts the body under great stress as it tries very hard to cope with everything. Just fruit and vegetable juices for a couple of days after a session will help the liver clean the system of the toxic chemicals more quickly. The liver will be in no condition to process any food for a few days, but as soon as it has thrown out the toxins nourishment is vital. The principle of 'starve the body, starve the cancer' is not a very sensible one. Starving the body beyond its capacity does not help cancer in the long run, though it may in the initial phase. You need to feed the body correctly to allow its sanogenetic powers to function.

Follow the precepts of Regimen Therapy (see chapter 7). In addition:
• Switch over to organic food, to minimise your intake of chemicals or pesticides that would ultimately lodge in the liver and impair its

biochemical reaction. Chemotherapy puts a great strain on the liver.
• Don't go on a low-protein diet. The body needs enzymes to carry out biochemical processes, including toxin elimination, and it gets these from protein. A body may cope with a strict vegetarian diet when it is healthy, but at times of serious illness such a regime is not helpful. A vegetarian diet for short periods is useful, but include soaked almonds, bean sprouts, butter, milk, cottage cheese, live yoghurt and whey for protein.
• Avoid alcohol, coffee, unknown herbal potions, very spicy, oily or deep fried foods, and canned products.
• Don't smoke.
• Drink a juice of carrot, apple, celery, ginger, mint leaves, 1–2 cloves of garlic and beetroot daily for a month and then every other day. The fruit and vegetable enzymes will activate the digestive organs and enable them to function better. The

vitamins and minerals get potentised as they are released from the vegetables.

• Drink 2 litres of water every day, particularly during chemotherapy or radiotherapy (water will help flush toxins through the system).

• Chawanprash or Bioprash (see page 220) is an Ayurvedic supplement with numerous ingredients that serve as a tonic or energy booster. It contains almonds and pistachios, so be careful if you have a nut allergy.

• Ask about infusions of vitamins like C and B_{12}, and the minerals calcium, magnesium and selenium. During and after chemotherapy the body gets depleted of essential nutrients, primarily due to liver toxicity and cellular malfunction, so supplements can be of great benefit.

• Antioxidants like vitamins A, C and E are useful in boosting the body's immune system.

Conventional treatments

There is no doubt that chemotherapy can sometimes suppress the growth of cancer cells, but at a heavy cost. The side effects of chemotherapy drugs are extreme: they damage the liver, kidneys and normal healthy tissues, and have a devastating effect on the immune system. If these side effects did not occur, then perhaps chemotherapy would be the best option. Work is being carried out on drugs that would target only cancer cells and produce minimum side effects. Such an approach would help the body tremendously.

The dose and duration of chemotherapy drugs do not necessarily have to be as much as is recommended in the pharmaceutical guidelines. They can be reduced provided they are supplemented by other therapies. If the reduced dose of chemotherapy is supported by diet, relaxation techniques, massages and infusions of vitamin C and minerals such as magnesium, calcium and selenium, then there are likely to be fewer side effects. Our experience shows that patients can go through the entire course without fatigue, loss of appetite, nausea, sickness and so on;

they remain symptom-free. Radiotherapy and surgery target the cancer growths directly if they are large enough, as they rely on growths being detected by scanning techniques. They are less appropriate for malignant cells too small to be identified or where cancer cells have spread around the body and developed secondaries.

Cancer is a very complicated area of medicine and the prognosis is always unsure. In the desire to help their patients, some doctors take the attitude: 'Throw everything on the wall and hope that something will stick. If the patients survive that's wonderful, but if they don't one may reasonably assume there was no hope for them anyway.' I am not sure I can agree with this approach, unless the cancer is so virulent or aggressive that there is nothing to be lost by trying anything. However, the choice should ultimately be the patient's, and clinics in some parts of the world, especially Mexico, offer a variety of non-conventional therapies that report success in some cases. These include fasting, coffee enemas, injections of apricots, seed extracts, various herbal preparations claimed to have anti-cancer properties, magnetic therapy and ozone/oxygen therapy.

Other beneficial treatments

• Meditation and yoga. Learn simple meditation techniques from a qualified teacher and practise regularly. If you can't find an instructor, practise the yogic *Shavasana* (see page 68). These techniques, with their emphasis on breathing and relaxation, calm the nervous system and slow down the body, which can help to decelerate the erratic division of cancer cells. A relaxed, stress-free outlook also gives more energy to your body to fight the disease.

• Neck and spine massage will improve blood flow to the pituitary and hypothalamus, the master centres for general well-being.

• Take conscious steps to relax: learn some yoga relaxation techniques and, when well enough, benefit from country walks.

facing surgery

If you prepare yourself for surgery physically as well as psychologically, you will reap the benefits of a faster recovery after the operation, enabling you to get back to your normal routine more quickly.

• Stick strictly to the Regimen Therapy (see chapter 7) for a few weeks before undergoing surgery and you will improve your body's healing power, drastically cutting the post-surgical recovery period. It will also help you lose weight if you need to: being overweight will not help your powers of recuperation.

• Build up your physical strength as best you can with massage and exercise, particularly if the surgery is to a joint or involves cutting muscle. This will help quicker rehabilitation afterwards. If you only start physiotherapy after surgery it will take weeks longer to build up the same strength. If you are having joint surgery, such as a hip replacement, talk to a qualified physiotherapist or osteopath about exercises that will not worsen your condition and be too painful.

• Try to balance your day by having an afternoon siesta, a short walk after dinner (10–15 minutes) and get to bed early. All this will contribute to your general energy. Needless to say, a daily yoga routine that includes relaxation in the Corpse Pose for stress management (see page 68) is very beneficial.

• Take 500 mg of vitamin C daily or eat a sweet citrus fruit. In ancient Persia and Moghul India, the juice of sweet lemons was a cure-all energy-boosting drink, and in traditional Indian medicine it is recommended for all recuperating patients (you will have to go to an Oriental grocer to find them). The sweet–sour–bitter aftertaste of this juice indicates the perfect balance nature has provided. If drunk in moderation, it will not produce the acidity that orange juice does, because its bitter alkaloids counteract the acid. I strongly recommend this for pre- and post-operative periods, recuperation from a debilitating condition (especially flu, food poisoning or diarrhoea, miscarriage etc.).

• Chawanprash – a multi-purpose Ayurvedic supplement with 28 herbs blended to create a perfect daily tonic – is an ancient formulation that helps digestion and liver functions, aids bowel movements, boosts circulation, increases energy and improves sleep. A tablespoon of this paste in conjunction with following my Regimen Therapy (see chapter 7) can really 'keep the doctor away'. Beware of some commercial preparations that may have excess ghee, honey, nuts etc.

After the operation:
• Eat foods that will help speed your recuperation, such as chicken broth for calcium and nutrients; carrot and celery juice for potassium (good for muscle tone); and coral calcium as a calcium supplement (see page 170).
• Take arnica to dissipate bruising.
• Resume exercise, such as gentle stretches and sedate swimming, as soon as you can.

> Try to balance your day by having an afternoon siesta, a short walk after dinner and get to bed early.

> Build up your physical strength as best you can with massage and exercise.

chapter 24
psychological health

What we eat and drink affects not only our physical well-being but our mental state – I always say 'mind over matter is matter undermined'. We all know that alcohol and recreational drugs cause major changes in our mood, our inhibitions and the way we see life, and we recognise the 'buzz' that too much strong coffee can give. Those who regularly drink excess coffee are short-tempered, tense, have panic attacks and a low tolerance level.

Food works on our minds in subtle yet wide-reaching ways. Not everyone reacts to food in the same way or to the same degree. Food intolerances can cause anxiety or depression as well as more physical reactions. There are people who become very shaky and nervous after eating mushrooms, while dairy (lactose) intolerance often results in a lack of concentration and even confusion. For more on food intolerances and allergies, see pages 197–8.

Basically there are two types of nervous reactions: depressive (depression, melancholia) and manic (anxiety, panic attacks, paranoia, hyperactivity). The causes of these are multifactorial and often stem from deep-seated psychological disturbances. Food can also trigger nervous reactions, as well as both ameliorating and exacerbating existing states of mind. Much research is being carried out into the remarkable ability of certain foods to affect the brain at a chemical level, for example raising serotonin levels to promote sleep, alter mood and release endorphins, the body's own guard against pain.

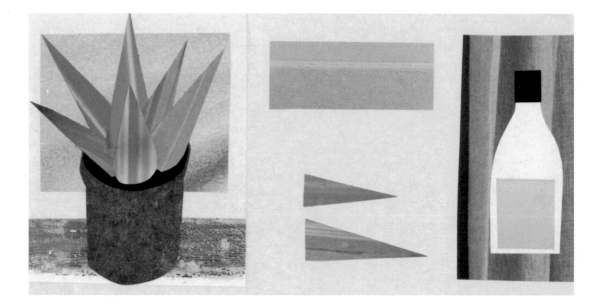

This is a very common psychological problem, and can also be part (either cause or effect) of many conditions: chronic fatigue syndrome, low blood pressure, Parkinson's disease, stroke, impotence or frigidity, infertility, diabetes and rheumatoid arthritis, to name just a few. It can be brought on by whiplash or traumatic brain injury, and there are many drugs of which depression is a recognised side effect, from betablockers (used to reduce high blood pressure) and anti-cholesterol drugs to antibiotics, painkillers, cortisone and other anti-inflammatory drugs.

Depression is often not properly diagnosed – just because you feel chronically tired, with low moods, doesn't necessarily mean you are clinically depressed. For true depression, anti-depressants have changed the scenario in recent years, but they should be used very cautiously, because of their addictiveness and other side effects, such as loss of appetite, impotence, weight gain etc. Being

aware of the depressant and energising effects of foods, however, can make a difference to any low mood.

Dietary guidance

Avoid:
- Alcohol.
- Yeast products (which will brew alcohol in the gut).
- Coffee.
- Chocolates, sweets and excess sugar in tea.
- Chamomile tea.

Eat the following foods, which can help to lift your mood:
- Carrot and ginger juice.
- Honey in milk or tea.
- Ginseng tea.
- Fenugreek leaves in cooking.
- Mildly spiced food (with black or red pepper or chillies).
- Aloe vera juice (see illustration opposite).
- More protein in diet.
- Soaked almonds or sweet almond oil in milk with honey.
- Olives.

Helpful nutritional supplements

- St John's wort.
- Chawanprash (an Ayurvedic supplement, see page 220).
- Multivitamins and minerals (but not on a long-term, uninterrupted basis).

Other beneficial treatments

- Psychological therapy.
- Homeopathy.
- Acupuncture.
- Therapeutic yoga.
- Meditation.

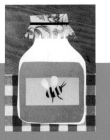

honey

Containing a combination of glucose and fructose, honey boosts energy and has many therapeutic properties. It soothes sore throats and acts as an expectorant, as well as having antiseptic qualities. Bee pollen (propolis) has medicinal uses, including promoting an anti-allergic reaction for the treatment of hay fever and eczema. It is a great alternative to sugar (which has depressive effects as soon as it is metabolised, leading to cravings and subsequent weight gain).

Stress is a factor in many health problems, from stomach ulcers and high blood pressure to psoriasis and depression. The reverse is also true: any serious, long-term or incurable illness, such as cancer, chronic fatigue syndrome, rheumatoid arthritis or Aids, is inevitably extremely stressful. Whatever the initial cause, it is all too easy to create a vicious circle, in which stress exacerbates the illness, which leads to greater stress and so on. It is important to recognise this as early as possible, and to seek help in reversing the cycle to become a virtuous circle.

Dietary guidance

Some foods may bring on a form of mania – hyperactivity – in susceptible children (see pages 81–2).

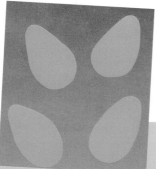

almonds

These nuts contain zinc, which may account for their use as an aphrodisiac, because zinc increases sperm production. The process of germination enriches the nuts with fresh protein, and soaked almonds are also full of essential amino acids and antioxidants. They improve the circulation of blood and almond oil is useful for regulating blood pressure.

Avoid foods that create the same symptoms in the body as stress: a racing heart, constricted blood vessels and tensed muscles. These include:
• Excess alcohol.
• Coffee and caffeine drinks.
• Ginger, garlic, chillies and highly spiced food.
• Sweets and sugary foods (especially in the evening, as sugar can set the brain racing and bring on insomnia).
• Excess salt, and salty foods like bacon, preserved fish and soy sauce.
• MSG (monosodium glutamate, a common flavour enhancer in Chinese food).
• Ginseng.

Drink plenty of water, as dehydration causes the heart to race and tenses up the muscles.

Several herbal teas, including mint, rose and chamomile, have a calming effect, as do the following foods:
• Watermelon, honeydew melon and squashes.
• Cucumber.
• Courgettes.
• Spring onions.
• Parsley.
• Summer berries.
• Live yoghurt and buttermilk.
• Sweet lime juice and elderflower cordial.

Chamomile, fennel, nettle and dandelion also help dilate constricted blood vessels.

Don't add to the strain on your body by eating lots of hard-to-digest foods, such as coarse, chewy meat and fatty foods.

Massage the neck and shoulders to improve blood and cerebrospinal fluid flow to the brain. This will supply extra oxygen to the hypothalamus and limbic systems (which control emotions) and calms them down. Non-competitive exercise is a good stress reliever, and take time out every day for some yoga or meditation (see chapter 7). Acupuncture, cranial osteopathy and homeopathy are all helpful aids to stress.

coping with a panic attack

A panic attack is characterised by hyperventilation (overfast breathing), a quickened heart beat, muscle tension (including in the jaws, which become very tight) and extreme stress. Blood pressure may rise, too.

Getting someone who is having a panic attack to breathe into a paper bag is simple and sensible. We exhale carbon dioxide, so breathing in carbon dioxide (from the bag) warns the brain of acute oxygen deficiency, and the heart and lungs are commanded to calm down as a defensive mechanism. As the heart slows down and the breathing rate drops, the panic attack abates. *Pranayama* (yogic breathing) or breath retention is extremely beneficial for the same reason. As soon as you hold your breath, the carbon dioxide level in the blood rises. In response the muscles relax and blood vessels dilate, so that the tissues of the heart, body and brain can quickly receive as much of whatever oxygen is available. The high concentration of carbon dioxide in the red blood cells is exchanged for oxygen very rapidly when you inhale.

The technique of *pranayama* is as follows: hold your breath for 15–20 seconds by squeezing your nostrils. Just when you think you are completely starved of air, open the nostrils gently, exhale and inhale just a small amount of air. Hold your breath again for 10–15 seconds and repeat the process. If you practise this when you are feeling calm, you'll find it comes naturally if you do experience a panic attack.

Alternatively, breath retention requires less practice. Inhale for three seconds, hold your breath for six seconds, then exhale for six seconds. Keep doing this for ten minutes.

EATING DISORDERS

There is a completely different way in which food and the mind interact, that of eating disorders such as anorexia nervosa and bulimia. Stress, insecurity, low self-esteem and other such distresses can manifest themselves in many different ways, from compulsive behaviour to self-harm, and including eating disorders.

With anorexia there is a constant fear or worry of putting on weight by eating certain things. An anorexic's view of her or his body becomes skewed, almost as if he or she were looking in a distorted fairground mirror. A minimal diet, devoid of protein, leads to deficiencies of fat-soluble vitamins such as vitamin D, essential for calcium absorption and vitamin E, necessary for hormonal functions. Anorexics, therefore, are prone to spontaneous fractures and to amenorrhoea (lack of menstrual periods), as well as the variety of ills associated with malnutrition. Anorexia can be life-threatening, with progressive symptoms including palpitations, kidney failure, ruptured spleen and cardiac arrest. Bulimia nervosa is a similarly severe eating disorder, but characterised by binge-eating alternating with vomiting. Because weight loss is less dramatic it can be harder to recognise.

My practical advice on nutritional help for anorexics and bulimics is given in Chapter 9, because these eating disorders are generally associated with teenage girls. However, boys and older adults are certainly not immune, and the guidance given on pages 87–9 applies to sufferers of both genders and all ages.

A point to remember is that anorexia and bulimia are adopted, not for comfort or pleasure, but by determination and willpower. They are a lifestyle choice. Although on the surface the focus is on food and diet, sufferers need more than guidance in nutrition. Such imbalances in self-perception need professional help. Find a psychiatrist sympathetic to natural methods of treatment.

epilogue

There was a time when malnutrition was the result of a bad diet due to a lack of sufficient food. Now malnutrition, at least in the prosperous West, stems from a bad diet due to too much of almost everything. While the poor in some parts of the world are afflicted by deficiency diseases and infections from bad hygiene, on the other side of the globe people are often eating a non-nutritious, over-refined diet by choice, and are suffering from a diet polluted by pesticides and chemicals. I wonder how many people, fifty years from now, will look back and wish they had treated their bodies to a healthy, nutritious diet? A lack of moderation, ignorance about what is good and bad for our bodies and the overpowering influence of the food industry means that all over the developed world people are suffering from nutrition-related illnesses.

If you read Eric Schlosser's *Fast Food Nation* (Penguin, 2001), you will surely get indigestion. This widely acclaimed book contains frightening revelations about the disastrous change in the eating habits of Americans, which has more recently spread to the rest of the Western world. As Schlosser reveals, the massive growth in the consumption of fast foods, hamburgers, fries and sodas has led to a devastating increase in obesity and food poisoning. A typical order of double cheeseburger and fries can contain up to 73 g of fat, more fat than ten milk shakes, while a regular can of soda contains the equivalent of 10 teaspoonfuls of sugar. As a result the USA has the highest obesity rate of any industrialised country in the world: over half its adults and a quarter of its children are categorised as obese. Obesity has been linked to heart disease, colon cancer, stomach cancer, breast cancer, diabetes, arthritis, high blood pressure, infertility and strokes. About 280,000 Americans die every year as a direct result of being overweight, and the epidemic is

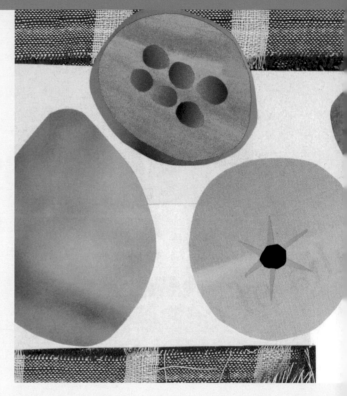

spreading worldwide. In Britain, the number of fast food restaurants has escalated dramatically over the last 20 years, and so has the obesity rate among adults. The British now eat more fast food than any other nation in western Europe.

Most fast food is delivered to the restaurant already frozen, canned, dehydrated or freeze-dried; the kitchen is merely the final stage in a vast and complex system of mass production. Poor-quality control results in frequent food poisoning. Schlosser points out that every day in the USA, roughly 200,000 people are taken ill with food-borne disease, 900 are taken to hospital and 14 die.

The food industry – which encompasses not only agriculture (or 'agribusiness'), food processing and retailing, but transport (think of all those Kenyan beans, Spanish tomatoes and coffee beans being shipped around the world), packaging and advertising – shapes the content of our larders

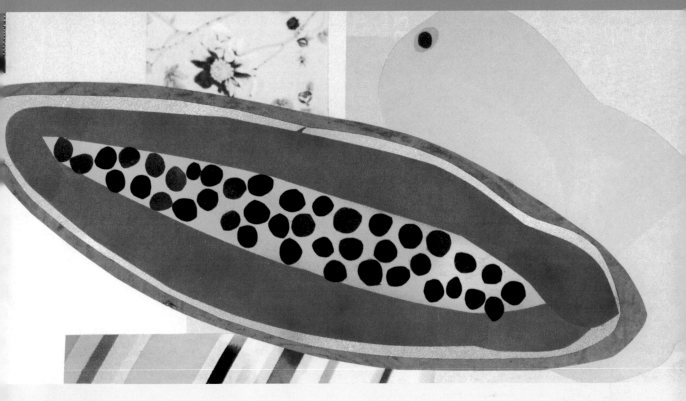

and fridges, and what we put on our tables. We have allowed ourselves to be conditioned to want the shiny, attractive and uniform over the well-raised and high-nutrient, to favour the fast and convenient over the good, and the exotic over the home-grown.

Schlosser also shows that children are specifically targeted in advertisements, especially the under eights, because they are the most susceptible and long-lasting. A survey of children's advertising in the European Union found that 95 per cent of food advertisements aimed at children encouraged them to eat foods high in sugar, salt and fat. Then riding on the very profitable coat-tails of the industry is the huge world of pharmaceuticals, which has made many fortunes from the rise in demand for antacids, vitamin and mineral supplements and quick cure-alls for ills that are of our own making. And yet … the food

industry argues that it is supplying what people want.

It may be difficult to see what an individual can do against the routine injection of hormones into livestock, the introduction of genetically modified crops on to the supermarket shelves and the endemic use of preservatives and additives, but there is a growing choice of alternatives, and the future is looking rosier than a decade ago. Organic food is becoming more widely available and we are hearing more about the success of small, caring food producers. If we raise the standards of what we require from food, good food could, in time, become the norm. If nobody buys fast food, there would be no profit in selling it. If we improved our health we will not need to spend so much money either directly on medication or indirectly on the health service. The voting power of our purses carries great weight.

Dr Ali's treatments

To arrange a medical consultation please contact:

Integrated Medical Centre
43 New Cavendish Street
London W1G 9TH
Telephone: 020 7224 5111
Fax: 020 7317 1600
www.dr-ali.co.uk

To order any of the products mentioned in the book or listed below please contact:

Integrated Health Products
43 New Cavendish Street
London W1G 9TH
Telephone: 020 7224 5141
Fax: 020 7224 3087
www.dr-ali.co.uk

Dr Ali's Arthritis Oil (joint oil)
Dr Ali's Bioenergy Tea
Dr Ali's Bioprash/Chawanprash
Dr Ali's Fasting Tea
Dr Ali's Gokhru Tea
Dr Ali's Junior Massage oil (sweet almond, eucalyptus and lavender)
Dr Ali's Lifestyle Oil
Dr Ali's Relaxation Tape
Dr Ali's Skin Oil
Dr Ali's Stomach Formula
Dr Ali's Winter Tea
Ayurvedic oil bath with specific medicated oil (removes inflammation of the joints, ligaments and tendons)
Bioflame Ayurvedic scalp massage oil
Bioliv
Bio Margosa Shampoo
Floral essences
Haldi
Neem Ayurvedic toothpaste

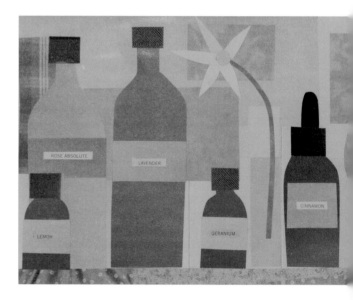

Previous books:
The Integrated Health Bible, ISBN 0 091 85626 4
Dr Ali's Ultimate Back Book, ISBN 0 091 88239 7
Therapeutic Yoga, ISBN 0 091 88514 0

index